T0201409

Making Sense of Medical Statistics

'This is an excellent introductory book for medical statistics. It's well written, easy to read, with some great examples of statistics in everyday clinical practice. The question and answer format is especially useful in reinforcing key concepts discussed in the chapter. There are lots of additional learning material included in the online resource for those seeking a more detailed understanding of the topic. The author is to be congratulated on making an important but difficult subject appear relatively straightforward and interesting to even the non-expert.'

Professor Paul Banaszkiewicz, Consultant Orthopaedic Surgeon North East NHS Surgical Centre (NENSC), Gateshead, UK, and Visiting Professor Northumbria University, Newcastle-upon-Tyne, UK

'An accessible book by a practising doctor, aimed at other doctors, which explains key statistical concepts in words and pictures. An excellent foundation for those seeking to understand the numbers in medical journal articles and quantitative reports.'

Professor Trish Greenhalgh, University of Oxford, UK

'The book provides a light-hearted introduction to the basic concepts in medical statistics. A couple of hundred pages long with short chapters, the book delivers with clear focus the key statistical concepts alongside some general knowledge to lighten what is sometimes a very arid subject. The description of concepts with graphs and figures support the visual learner. I thoroughly enjoyed the quick questions presented alongside the description of concepts to test understanding, with the answers at the end of chapter which linked to bullet point summaries, help to consolidate the concepts covered. I thought it was an excellent way for someone to start on their path to understanding this area. Finally, I particularly appreciated the last chapter with its focus on the work by our dear friend Doug Altman.'

Professor Rafael Perera, Professor of Medical Statistics, University of Oxford, UK

'Statistics forms the starting point for evidence based medicine, though most medics would argue that their own statistical awareness is still near the starting point! This book eases you into the awesome, exciting, exhilarating world of statistics, and makes you understand just how cool it really is. It will unleash your inner statistician that no-one knew existed – especially you!'

Professor Dan Perry, Children's Orthopaedic Surgeon and Fellow of Wolfson College, University of Oxford, UK

Making Sense of Medical Statistics

Munier Hossain
MBBS, FRCSGlag, FRCSG (Tr & Orth), PGCE, MSc (Orth Eng), MSc (Oxon), FHEA
Consultant Orthopaedic Surgeon
United Lincolnshire Hospitals NHS Trust

Illustrations and formatting by
Inda Zubir
B.Sc (Hons), M.Arch, RIBA III

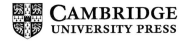

CAMBRIDGE
UNIVERSITY PRESS

CAMBRIDGE
UNIVERSITY PRESS

University Printing House, Cambridge CB2 8BS, United Kingdom

One Liberty Plaza, 20th Floor, New York, NY 10006, USA

477 Williamstown Road, Port Melbourne, VIC 3207, Australia

314–321, 3rd Floor, Plot 3, Splendor Forum, Jasola District Centre,
New Delhi – 110025, India

103 Penang Road, #05–06/07, Visioncrest Commercial, Singapore 238467

Cambridge University Press is part of the University of Cambridge.

It furthers the University's mission by disseminating knowledge in the pursuit of education, learning, and
research at the highest international levels of excellence.

www.cambridge.org
Information on this title: www.cambridge.org/9781108978156
DOI: 10.1017/9781108973663

© Munier Hossain 2021

This publication is in copyright. Subject to statutory exception and to the provisions of relevant collective
licensing agreements, no reproduction of any part may take place without the written permission of
Cambridge University Press.

First published 2021
Reprinted 2022

Printed in the United Kingdom by TJ Books Limited, Padstow Cornwall

A catalogue record for this publication is available from the British Library.

ISBN 978-1-108-97815-6 Paperback

Cambridge University Press has no responsibility for the persistence or accuracy of URLs for external or
third-party internet websites referred to in this publication and does not guarantee that any content on such
websites is, or will remain, accurate or appropriate.

In memory of

Mr Ismail Hossain BA, LLB, Dip Air and Space Law, LLM (McGill)

List of Contents

Online content which can be found at www.cambridge.org/medicalstatistics

Preface

What is the point of another book on medical statistics? That is a question I have grappled with for some time. The more so when one considers that the subject is so well served by the most eminent of statisticians. I am not a statistician by training and only have an amateur interest in this subject. What do I hope to contribute to this crowded field?

I have been trying to learn and teach medical statistics for nearly a decade. Over the years I have come to appreciate the difficulty my peers face when trying to learn it. The available books mostly aim to turn health professionals into budding statisticians. They are full of complex formulas and problems, but health professionals don't need to be statisticians, nor do they need to learn any equations. Rather, they need a working understanding. Health professionals need to understand the principles of medical statistics so that they can understand what questions to ask, when to ask, which tests to employ to get the answers and how to interpret the results correctly.

I tried to make statistics learning fun, interactive and easy. The concepts of statistics can be difficult to understand from words alone. Hence, I wanted to make use of illustrations to communicate with my readers and make statistics learning easier. I also wanted to see if I could employ some of the principles of adult learning, which I use in my courses, directly into a book. This book does not offer an in-depth look at medical statistics. The chapters are bite-sized in length so that readers do not lose grip of their attention span. My emphasis has been on teaching the concepts and encouraging the learner to think and ask questions along the way. Thus, the book is intended as a guide, not a preacher. I hope it will provide the reader with enough of a foundation to find his/her way through the maze of medical statistics.

I wanted the book to be relevant to medics' working life and their exam preparation. That is why, in addition to the print version, we included online material that contains single best answers in the format of professional exams, references and resources for further learning as well as links to statistical software and questions to practice data analysis.

Ultimately, this book is about you, the learner. If you have benefitted, please let us know. If you find mistakes, please leave us feedback. If you have suggestions for improvement, please get in touch. We would be delighted to acknowledge your contribution in future editions.

You can get in touch via medstatsfeedback@gmail.com

Acknowledgements

I want to start by thanking God Almighty for everything. On a more prosaic level, there are a lot of people without whose help and support this book would never have seen the light of the day. I am genuinely grateful to you all. Of those who deserve a special mention, let me start by thanking my parents first. My wife and daughter have been my biggest supporters. Thank you for your patience and understanding. My parents-in-law also offered me constant encouragement.

My teachers at the Centre for Evidence-Based Medicine, University of Oxford taught me the craft of medical statistics and the art of effective teaching. The ideas expounded in this book are an extension of what I learnt in Oxford.

Jean Williams and Kim O'Neill of Postgraduate Centre, Ysbyty Gwynedd offered me the first platform to teach medical statistics. Paul Banaszkiewicz and Sattar Alshryda asked me to write a chapter on medical statistics for the British Orthopaedic Association Wikipaedics project that, although unsuccessful, sparked my earliest interest in writing this book. Paul has also been a rock of support behind this project from day one. Paul Banaszkiewicz, Vijay Bhalaik, Badri Narayan, David Green, Rajesh Power and Hidayah Ma offered helpful comments on the earliest draft. Nik Abidin's suggestions helped me to improve my punctuation and grammar. Daniel Green and Rebecca Simpson, both academic statisticians from the University of Sheffield, diligently went through the draft copy. Their input was crucial in correcting mistakes and improving the contents. Sir Iain Chalmers, despite his hectic schedule, went through some chapters in great detail, pointed out errors and suggested improvements. I am also grateful to Professor Trish Greenhalgh for her kind endorsement. Inda Zubir, a talented young architect and graphic artist, took my raw diagrams and turned them into superb illustrations. She also did the formatting. The lion's share of the credit for the visual appeal of this book goes to Inda. A very special thanks to her.

I am indebted to the Editorial Committee of the Bone and Joint Journal and the Cochrane Collaboration for allowing me to reproduce some copyrighted figures. Numerous images have been reproduced courtesy of the Creative Commons licence. I am grateful for and acknowledge their contribution to keeping the frontiers of knowledge open. I am thankful to the Cambridge University Press and especially Nick Dunton who was brave enough to bank on an unknown author of no proven pedigree in a crowded and well-catered-for field. Jessica Papworth, Katy Nardoni, Olivia Boult, Bethan Lee and many others have worked hard behind the scenes to make this book a reality. My thanks to them all.

Finally, all the delegates who attended my courses over the years, your appreciation and feedback spurred me on.

How to Get the Most Out of This Book

Throughout the book we tried to make learning fun, relevant, interactive and visual. Keeping in mind the differing needs of learners we tried to cater to everyone's needs by dividing each chapter into different levels of learning. Before you delve into them it may help to get familiar with the icons displayed in each chapter. Here is a road-map for the journey ahead.....

What's the sidebar for?

There is a sidebar in every page with the following icons:

 Every chapter starts with defined learning outcomes

 and ends with important take home messages.

Your core learning content is in between these two icons. If interested, you will find additional learning material further afield...

 A more advanced Bonus section that may contain formulas!

 This is the section with answers to all the brain-teasers.

There is even more material online.

 Single Best Answer questionniares in the format of professional exams.

 Software and practice corner with questions and solutions, to get you up to speed with data analysis.

 References and recommended reading.

List of useful books, free statistical software, helpful webpages and YouTube videos.

There is something for everyone. Happy reading!!

Did You Know?

Interesting anecdotes to spice up your reading!

Bullet Points

Key information is emphasised to help reinforce your memory.

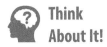 Think About It!

A bit of brainwork to fire up the neurons and support your learning.

CHAPTER 1

Medicine and Numbers
Where Is the Connection?

[…] for complete initiation as an efficient citizen of one of the new great complex world-wide States that are now developing, it is as necessary to be able to compute, to think in averages and maxima and minima, as it is now to be able to read and write.

H.G. Wells

 Learning Outcomes

We shall discuss the following material in this chapter:
• Why physicians need to study medical statistics
• The utility of descriptive statistics
• The utility of inferential statistics

Did You Know?

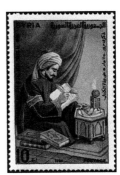

© Unknown author/ public domain [1].

Figure 1.1 The scholar depicted in this Syrian postage stamp is **Abu Yusuf Al Kindi** (801 – 873), an Arab mathematician and polymath. He is credited with making one of the earliest known statistical analysis in his treatise *On Deciphering Cryptographic Messages* [2].

Medical Statistics : A Modern-Day Crystal Ball

At first glance, medicine and numbers may appear far too much apart, but a closer inspection will tell a different story. In days gone by, people turned to ball-gazers in search of answers for health, happiness and future. We now live in a universe of big data. Where crystal balls, distant stars or dried bones once conspired to rule upon citizens' lives, information now reigns supreme. A random set of numbers is no good until we apply the powerful tool of data analysis. It is the best means we currently have of making a meaningful pattern out of a group of random numbers. The insight we gain helps us to make predictions for the future. Statistics is our modern-day crystal ball: it is the collection and analysis of data that is our window to the past, interpreter of the present and guide to the future. With the widespread availability of statistical software, the calculation of statistics is no longer complicated. The key to getting the right answer from our crystal ball is to appreciate when to choose which statistics and to recognise the nuances of the reply.

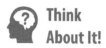

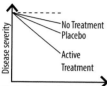

Figure 1.2 Comparison of disease severity between no treatment and active treatment [3]. © BMC Medical Research Methodology, CC BY 2.0 .

What does Figure 1.2 suggest?

Apart from numbers, can descriptive statistics be conveyed in any other fashion?

What is the limitation of descriptive statistics?

Why don't we discuss uncertainty while relaying descriptive statistics?

Why Do We Need to Study Medical Statistics?

Nobody expects a physician to study medical statistics to become a fully fledged statistician, although no one will stop you. Yet, a fundamental understanding of statistics is essential for all physicians in our everyday practice. In our everyday lives, we research every product we buy, compare ratings, look at reviews and feedback before making decisions. The modern man or woman makes a well-informed decision before committing to a product. Medicine is no different. We need to learn medical statistics so that we can make informed decisions about patient care.

Statistics gives us the tools to find a pattern from a random set of numbers borne out of observations, experiments and trials, and to communicate the results meaningfully. Understanding this common language allows both the researcher and the audience to make sense of the numbers. Informed decision-making is only possible if we can understand what kind of test was performed, why it was performed, what was the size and effect of an intervention, as well as its significance. Understanding this will allow us to differentiate between hype and truth.

Descriptive Statistics: Seeing the Wood and the Trees

A useful function of medical statistics (Figure 1.3) is to **describe** the data observed in an experiment or trial in a condensed format and relay the information in a way that is understood by readers. This part of medical statistics is known as **descriptive statistics**. Descriptive statistics help us to make sense out of the confusion of random numbers.

For example, if we measure weight, we shall employ descriptive statistics to understand as well as inform the reader about the average weight, the distribution from the lightest to the heaviest, and the most frequent weight observed etc.

Here is an example from a recent study where the authors wished to investigate the prevalence of musculoskeletal injury (MSK-I) among athletes [4]:

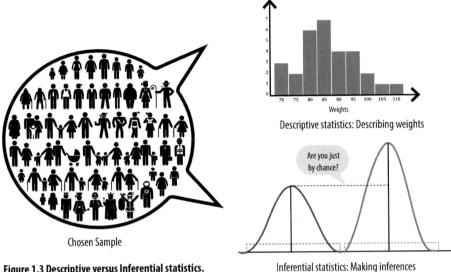

Descriptive statistics: Describing weights

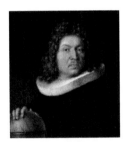

Figure 1.3 Descriptive versus Inferential statistics.

Inferential statistics: Making inferences

In this cross-sectional observational study, 627 athletes from rugby (n = 225), soccer (n = 172), combat sports (n = 86), handball (n = 82) and water polo (n = 62) were recruited at different sports training centres and competitions. The mean age was 25 ± 6 years, and 60% of the athletes were male [...]. The MSK-I prevalence among all athletes was 76%, with 55% of MSK-I occurring in a joint, 48% occurring in a muscle and 30% being tendinopathy, and 19% of athletes had three investigated injuries. There was a predominance of joint injury in combat sports athletes (77%), muscle injury in handball athletes (67%) and tendinopathy in water polo athletes (52%).

Inferential Statistics

When we observe a characteristic, it is seldom possible to investigate everyone with it. Instead, we choose a representative sample. Therefore, we need tools to be able to infer from our limited observational values to the unknown but much larger total population. By employing the tools available in **inferential statistics**, we can predict how everyone else with the same characteristic is likely to behave.

We can estimate the unknown population parameter, the plausible range of this parameter, if it differs between two

Did You Know?

© Public domain [5]

Figure 1.4 Random events play a large role in our lives. **The law of large numbers** is central to understanding probability. It was first described by a Swiss mathematician **Jacob Bernoulli**(1655–1705). It states that if the same experiment is repeated manifold, the average of results gets closer to the real mean.

Bullet Points

Descriptive statistics:

to summarise and present the observations.

Inferential statistics:

-to make inferences about the larger population from the available observations.

-to estimate the unknown population parameter.

-to calculate the plausible range of the effect size.

-to estimate the probability that differences in observations might be due to chance.

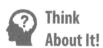

Think About It!

What is the difference between descriptive and inferential statistics?

populations, the probability that chance or random variation might have affected the results, and how a particular characteristic is influenced by others, etc. Since we make inferences from a limited sample to a larger population, there is **always** a degree of **uncertainty** in **inferential statistics**. If we take the example of measuring weights, we shall employ inferential statistics to help us infer regarding the likely average weight of the whole population of interest, who is most at risk of obesity, and what we can do to prevent it etc.

For example, let's refer back to the above study [4]. Ideally, to investigate the prevalence of MSK-I one should ask every athlete if they have ever had MSK-I but this is not feasible. Therefore, the authors recruited a sample and recorded their observations. From the observations, the authors were able to make inferences. Here is more from the same abstract [4]:

> Age (≥ 30 years) was positively associated with joint (OR = 5.2 and 95% CI = 2.6–10.7) and muscle (OR = 4.9 and 95% CI = 2.4–10.1) injuries and tendinopathy (OR = 4.1 and 95% CI = 1.9–9.3) [...] The analysis of associated factors (epidemiological, clinical and sports profiles) and the presence of MSK-I in athletes suggests an approximately 4-5-fold increased risk for athletes ≥ 30 years of age.

The authors undertook statistical tests and were able to conclude that age ≥ 30 was the most important risk factor for MSK-I. They also calculated the likely magnitude of the risk (OR: Odds Ratio). These tests allowed them to make educated guesses regarding the unknown population parameter that we would likely find if we studied the whole population. They also calculated the accuracy of their estimate (95% CI: Confidence Interval), and by calculating the p-value, the authors were able to estimate the probability that the observed differences between different groups of athletes could be affected by chance alone.

The first step in our journey to understanding medical statistics is to appreciate that there are differences in individual characteristics that dictate what kind of statistical tests we perform. Let's begin in the next chapter.

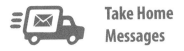

Take Home Messages

- Learning medical statistics enables us to:-

- Make sense of data.
- Communicate results effectively.
- Understand the language of researchers.
- Make up our minds regarding the effectiveness of an intervention.
- Be an evidence-informed physician.

- Medical statistics is divided into two branches: descriptive statistics and inferential statistics.

- Descriptive statistics are necessary to summarise and present collected data.

- Inferential statistics allow us to make inferences from the collected data about the population at large even though we may not have observed the whole population of interest.

Questions & Answers

Q: What does Figure 1.2 suggest?

A: This graph plots pre- and post-treatment disease state on the *x*-axis and disease severity on the *y*-axis. One can conclude that patients in the trial got better regardless of treatment. However, the magnitude of improvement was highest with active treatment, followed by that of placebo effect compared to no treatment alone. Therefore, when we observe improvement in disease activity, it is essential to appreciate that patients can get better without any treatment in the natural course of events. However, the margin of difference between the therapeutic effect, the placebo effect, and spontaneous improvement due to the natural history of the disease may not be the same. We plan to revisit the placebo effect in Chapter 9.

Q: Apart from numbers, can descriptive statistics be relayed in any other fashion?

A: Yes, descriptive statistics are often relayed visually by bar charts, pie-charts, histograms etc.

Q: What is the limitation of descriptive statistics?

A: The limitation of descriptive statistics is that we cannot make any inferences from the results or understand the underlying issues. For example, looking back at the previous study we understand that joint injury was most common and that athletes engaged in combat sports, handball and water polo were most susceptible to injury in their sample. We do not know if the results might be true for the general population [4].

Q: Why don't we discuss uncertainty while relaying descriptive statistics?

A: Descriptive statistics are only a summary of the observed sample; there is no uncertainty in this information.

Q: What is the difference between descriptive and inferential statistics?

A: Descriptive statistics are a summary of the observed sample. Inferential statistics attempt to make inferences from the results of the available sample to the broader population.

CHAPTER 2

Measuring a Variable
Why Eye Colour and Height Are Different

The law of anomalous numbers is thus a general probability law of widespread application.

Frank Benford

🎯 Learning Outcomes

We shall discuss the following material in this chapter:
- What is a variable
- The different types of variables
- The difference between a sample and a population

What Is a Variable, and What Are the Different Types?

A variable is a measurable characteristic (age, weight, height, sex, etc.) (Figure 2.2). The first step in clinical research is to identify a pertinent 'variable' of interest and to observe it. These observations subsequently form the dataset.

All variables are not the same. It is vital to appreciate the difference in variables as this difference dictates how we measure them and what type of statistical test we can perform. Variables are of two types (Figure 2.3).

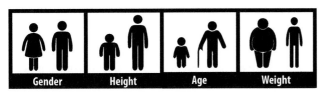

Figure 2.2 Example of variables.

Did You Know?

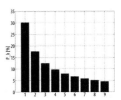

© Gknor, Public domain [1].

Figure 2.1 Benford's law states that the leading digit in naturally occurring numbers is most frequently small, number one occurs around 30% of the time, number nine only 5%. The reach of this law is universal, from celestial bodies to mundane stock prices. It has been rumoured, but not confirmed, that the US tax agency utilises this law to catch tax-evaders! Benford's law also rules the digital universe. You can use it to catch Twitter bots, or fake digital images [2].

Numerical variable		Categorical variable		
Measuring weight	Counting numbers	Tick box	Grading obesity	Iris colour
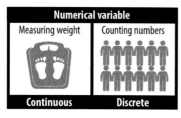		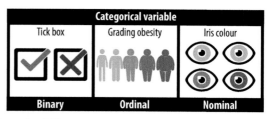		
Continuous	Discrete	Binary	Ordinal	Nominal

Figure 2.3 Types of variables.

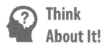

Think About It!

Can you think of a study where we would include the whole population of interest?

Why is it important to appreciate the differences in variables?

Can variables be treated interchangeably?

How is information on continuous variables relayed in Table 2.1 and why?

Numerical variables can be discrete or continuous:
- **Discrete**: counts, e.g. number of adults, days of the week etc.
- **Continuous**: height, blood pressure etc.

Categorical data can be categorised into groups; these can be either binary (of two types) or more than two types:
- **Binary**: smoker or non-smoker, dead or alive.

> 2 types: nominal or ordinal:
- **Nominal**: categories are not in order: eye colour, blood group.
- **Ordinal**: categories are in order: patient satisfaction, tumour stage.

Variable	Rugby (n = 225)	Soccer (n = 172)
Age (years)		
<20	28 (12.4)	58 (33.7)
20-24	96 (42.8)	47 (27.3)
25-29	64 (28.4)	33 (19.2)
>30	37 (16.4)	34 (19.8)
Sex		
Female	160 (71.1)	0
Male	65 (28.9)	172 (100.0)
Height (cm)		
<165	89 (39.6)	5 (2.9)
165-174	72 (32.0)	45 (26.2)
175-184	49 (21.8)	72 (41.9)
>185	15 (6.6)	50 (29.1)
Alcohol consumption		
No	66 (29.3)	95 (55.2)
Yes	159 (70.7)	77 (44.8)

Table 2.1 Rugby versus soccer players, from Goes et al. © BMC Musculoskeletal disorders, reproduced with CC Licence [3].

Let's look at the table above (Table 2.1) [3]. The variables reported here are age, sex, height and alcohol consumption. What type of variables have the authors presented in this table? Why have these been presented in this fashion, can you think of alternate ways of presenting data? Could data on alcohol consumption be presented in any other way?

A Sample or a Population?

If one is interested in a particular variable, then everyone who has that variable should be observed. In reality, this is not feasible. Therefore, researchers settle for a carefully chosen smaller group: a '**sample**'. In designing a study or a trial, the researcher hopes that the observed 'sample' is representative of the larger group (Figure 2.4). The larger group is known as the '**population**' and includes **everyone who has the variable of interest**.

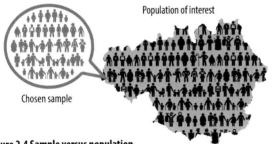

Figure 2.4 Sample versus population.

We make a lot of calculations from the data gathered and summarise the results. One measure of such calculation is known as the '**sample mean**'. We represent mean by the symbol $\bar{x}$. We measured the sample mean, but we aimed to estimate the population mean, which we do not know. The unknown population parameter which we hope to guess by estimating the sample mean is known as the '**population mean**' and it is indicated by μ.

How accurately our sample mean represents the population mean is dependent on how closely our chosen sample represents the population of interest. **The sample mean will vary** depending on the sample chosen and the precision of measurement, but the **population mean** will remain **constant**.

Now that we understand the differences between variables, and that of a sample and the population, let's learn how to collect data and present them in the next chapter!

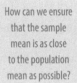

Think About It!

How can we ensure that the sample mean is as close to the population mean as possible?

Bullet Points

Variable:

a measurable characteristic of interest

Population:

everyone with the variable of interest

Sample:

a chosen section of the population; may or may not be representative of the population

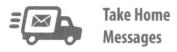 **Take Home Messages**

- A variable is a characteristic of interest.

- Variables are numerical or categorial.

- Numerical variables can be discrete or continuous.

- Categorical variables can be binary, nominal or ordinal.

- The population includes everyone with the variable of interest.

- A sample is a portion of the population that we studied.

- There is a difference between the population mean and the sample mean.

- The proximity between the sample mean and the population mean is dependent on how closely the sample represents the population and how accurate we are in our measurement.

Questions & Answers

Q: Can you think of a study where we would include the whole population of interest?

A: National Census is an observational study where we investigate the whole population of interest.

Q: Why is it important to appreciate the differences in variables?

A: It is essential to appreciate the differences in variables because each variable has its own characteristic behaviour. We know about the frequency distribution of different variables in the population. Hence, we are familiar with their respective expected frequencies and distributions. This distribution dictates the type of statistical tests we can perform to search for uncharacteristic behaviour that may be 'statistically significant'. These tests are crucial if we are to make valid inferences regarding the broader population.

Q: Can variables be treated interchangeably?

A: Yes; in Table 2.1, authors observed age and height, which are both continuous numerical variables but converted them into categorical types. Transforming data in this way may affect the variation found in the original data. Nevertheless, it is often undertaken to help interpret data or to produce statistics (for example, to determine odds ratios or relative risk).

Q. How is information on continuous variables relayed in Table 2.1 and why?

A: Age and height are both numerical and continuous variables. In Table 2.1, the authors displayed them as categorical variables. They divided the participants into four different age groups and height categories. This categorisation was done for the sake of convenience to help with data presentation and analyses.

Q: How can we ensure that the sample mean is as close to the population mean as possible?

A: We need to ensure that the chosen sample is as representative of the population as possible. The simplest way to ensure this is to have a sample that is as large as possible and is also representative of the variables of interest. Sample size by itself is not the sole indicator of representativeness.

CHAPTER 3

Summarising Data
Communicating Easily

A want of the habit of observing conditions and an inveterate habit of taking averages are each of them often equally misleading.

Florence Nightingale

Did You Know?

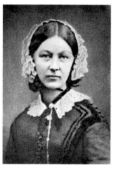

© Public domain [1].

Figure 3.1 Florence Nightingale **OM, RRC, DStJ** (1820–1910), was not only a pioneering nurse, she was also a ground-breaking statistician. She was the first female member of the Royal Statistical Society. During the Crimean war she used statistical analyses to improve the treatment of the wounded. On returning from the war, she pioneered the use of infographics to present data: the **'polar area diagram'** [2].

 Learning Outcomes

We shall discuss the following material in this chapter:
• Measures of central tendency
• The difference between mean, median and mode
• Measures of spread: range, interquartile range
• What is a percentile
• What is an outlier, and how do we display it

Making Sense of Data Chaos

When we first gather data, it is just a collection of apparently random numbers. How can we find the hidden pattern? Let's go to a swimming pool and find out.

There, we meet a group of youngsters enjoying swimming; we ask ten of them how old they are. Here are their ages in years:

7, 9, 9, 10, 10, 10, 10, 11, 11, 13

How can we relay this information in a format that is easier to understand? How can we summarise the numbers so that we can characterise this group?

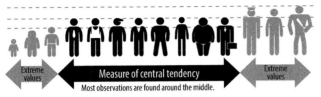

Figure 3.2 Distribution of height measurement, common and rare values.

One useful marker is the **measure of central tendency**. Central tendency is where we find most of the values; extreme values are obviously much less common. A measure of central tendency is useful to understand where the **majority** of **data** values can be found (Figure 3.2). Three commonly used measures to identify central tendency are mean, median and mode.

The measure of central tendency is a *point* estimate (a single value) that represents the *peak* of data in a symmetric distribution. It does not give us any information about the spread of data (Figure 3.3).

Mean: this is the mathematical average, a value that we are familiar with, a sum of all the data values divided by the number of data values. Looking back at our young swimmers:

The sum of their age is =
7+9+9+10+10+10+10+11+11+13 = 100

There are ten swimmers. The mean age
of our swimmers is 100÷10 = **10**

Median: to calculate the median value we first need to arrange the data in sequential order, the median is the value in the middle. In this case, there are ten observations; therefore, the median value is the sum of the fifth (10) and the sixth (10) observation divided by 2 = **10**.

If there were nine swimmers, the median age would be the age of the fifth swimmer. The median value equally splits the data into two halves. The weakness of this measure is that the median does not take account of other scores. Even if those scores were markedly different, if the middle score remained the same then the median would remain unaffected. This is advantageous when there are extreme values (outliers) in the dataset.

Did You Know?

The legend goes that during the Peloponnesian War (431–404 BC), fought between the armies of Sparta and Athens, the Athenians were able to correctly calculate the height of the ladder needed to scale the Platean walls by counting the number of bricks in sections of wall, calculating the mode value and multiplying it by the height of the bricks to determine the likely wall height [3].

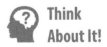

Think About It!

What is the advantage and disadvantage of using the mean value as a measure of central tendency?

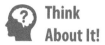

Think About It!

Why is mode the most suitable as a measure of central tendency for categorical variables?

Mode: the mode is the most frequent value, which in this case is **10**. Note that a dataset may contain multiple mode values or no mode value at all. Let us observe the age of another group of swimmers: 7,9,9,10,10,11,12,13.

Here ages 9 and 10 are both observed twice and would represent mode, or none if all the values occurred only once.

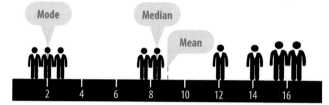

Figure 3.3 Mean, median and mode of weight illustrated with example. (Mean weight is 8.89 stones, median weight is 8 stones and mode is 2 stones).

Why is the mode value not suitable for numerical variables?

Why Do We Have Different Measures of Central Tendency and Which One Should I Choose?

We have different measures because each serves a different purpose, we cannot use any one of them universally. Often, it is the type of variable observed that dictates which one measure is the most suitable one. The mean is often the best measure for a numerical variable, although this is not always the best. Mean works best when data has a predictable and symmetric distribution, *we shall learn about data distribution in Chapter 5*. When this is not the case, the median is the preferred measure.

What does a large spread tell you about data?

What about Categorical Variables?

Can you think of a situation where measures of central tendency might be redundant?

Ordinal: Let us consider our young swimmer buddies. We asked them how satisfied they were with the day's swimming activity on a scale of 0–10, 0 being thoroughly dissatisfied and 10 being complete satisfaction. The scores were as follows: 4 (1), 5 (1), 6 (4), 7 (3), 8(1).

What is the advantage of using the median value?

Even though numbers were used, it was not an interval rating scale. The difference between age 7–8 and 8–9 is the same but the difference between ratings 1–2 and 3–4 is not the same. We cannot calculate the mean value of this rating. We could use the mode or the median as the measure of central tendency. Both are 6. The young swimmers appear, on average, happy with the day's activity.

Nominal: What if we want to know the blood group of the swimmers?

O +ve (2), O -ve (2), A +ve (5), AB+ve (1)

We cannot calculate the mean value. The observations do not have any order, and the median value cannot be calculated either. The mode would be our choice to indicate that A+ve was the most common blood type.

Bullet Points

Sample mean is indicated by the symbol $\bar{x}$.

Population mean is indicated by the symbol μ.

Measures of Spread

We met a group of swimmers, and we were curious about their age. We made enquiries, constructed a dataset, and relayed a bit of information about the data to the reader using measures of central tendency. We now understand that the swimmers are on **average, ten years** old. The average is just a single number (point estimate) and does not relay the full story. Who was the youngest, who was the oldest, how variable were the ages, what was the age difference between them?

We have no idea about any of this information. We do not know how representative the mean is of the dataset and what was the **variability** of the dataset. Therefore, more information is required to complete our understanding of the young swimmers' age.

Measures of spread give us some additional information. Similar to measures of central tendency, we can communicate measures of spread using several different values.

Range: the range is the difference between the highest and the lowest value. The age range of our swimmers is six, the youngest being seven and the oldest being thirteen years of age. The range is a simple and intuitive measure of spread but gives very little information, especially if there are extreme values in the dataset. We need other measures.

Interquartile range (IQR): a quartile divides the data into a quarter. To calculate the IQR, we count the number of observations. We had ten young swimmers; we need to divide this number by four. The *first* quartile is 10÷4 = the

Think About It!

'There was a *bi-modal age distribution of* [humeral shaft fracture]' [4]. What did the authors mean by the term 'bi-modal'?

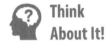

When would you consider IQR to be a better indicator of measure of spread compared to the range?

Bullet Points

Sample mean is indicated by the symbol $\bar{x}$.

Population mean is indicated by the symbol μ.

Inter Quartile Range (IQR):

upper quartile- lower quartile (i.e., middle 50% of data, it avoids both too large or too small extremes).

Percentile:

another measure of data spread, divides data into 100 equal groups. Twentieth percentile means 20% of data are below and 80% above this threshold. **IQR** is the data spread between the **75th** and the **25th percentile**.

Outlier:

an outlier is an extreme value in a dataset. If there is an extremely small or large value it will affect some of the measures. There is an outlier in figure 3.4 in group B, marked with a circle, note the score compared to the rest of the group. *We shall learn more about outliers in Chapter 5.*

2.5th observation. The *third* quartile is 2.5 × 3 = the 7.5th observation. The **IQR** is the *range* between upper quartile: Q3 - lower quartile: Q1. We sum the second and the third observation and divide by two (9+9 = 18÷2 = 9), our *first* quartile value is 9. We sum the seventh and the eigth observation and divide by two (10+11 = 21÷2 = 10.5), our *third* quartile value is 10.5.

The **IQR** is the *range* between *Q3 - Q1 =* **10.5 - 9.**

IQR is less affected by extreme values and is the preferred indicator of data spread when extreme values are present in the dataset. If a dataset has extreme values the distribution becomes skewed or nonsymmetric.

Nonsymmetric data are graphically **presented** in a **box and whisker plot** (Figure 3.4). The horizontal line inside the box represents the **median**; the lower and upper borders of the box represent the 25th and the 75th percentiles, respectively; the **whiskers** represent data range, excluding outliers (> 1.5-times the IQR below the first or above the third quartile). The circle represents extreme values or **outliers**. Authors compared the quality of life via the Toronto Extremity Salvage Score (TESS) after lower extremity amputation for bone or soft-tissue tumours. The figure suggests that TESS differed by amputation level, with poorer scores at higher levels in general.

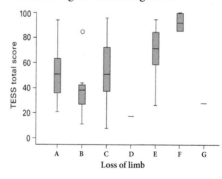

Figure 3.4 Box and whisker plot. Reproduced with permission and © of The British Editorial Society of Bone & Joint Surgery [5].

Measures of central tendency and spread are useful for a broad overview of data but may not always be adequate. Let us learn in the next chapter why we need more measures to describe data variation.

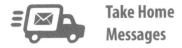

Take Home Messages

- There are two types of point estimates: measures of central tendency and measures of spread.

- There are three types of measures of central tendency: mean, median and mode.

- Mean is the arithmetic average and is useful for summarising symmetric data.

- Median is the middle observation and is useful when data includes outliers.

- Mode is the most frequent observation and is useful for summarising categorical data.

- Range and interquartile range are both measures of spread.

- Range is the difference between the highest and the lowest data values.

- Interquartile range contains the middle 50% of data.

- Interquartile range is the spread of data between the 75th and the 25th percentile.

- The interquartile range is useful for describing data with outliers.

- A box and whisker plot is employed to display the median and the interquartile range.

- An outlier is an extremely low or high value compared to the rest of the dataset.

- Outliers affect data distribution and make it nonsymmetric.

Questions & Answers

Q: What is the advantage and disadvantage of using the mean value as a measure of central tendency?

A: Of all the measures of central tendency, the mean value is the most intuitive and the most sensitive. Its calculation includes every observation in the dataset. However, the disadvantage of using the mean as a measure of central tendency in the presence of an outlier is that outliers can unduly influence the mean value and give a misleading representation of the central tendency. We shall learn more about such situations later.

Q: What is the advantage of using the median value?

A: The median value is not affected by outliers or skewed data. It is the preferred measure when data have outliers.

Q: Why is the mode most suitable as a measure of central tendency for categorical variables?

A: Mode gives information regarding the most common category. Mean is not computable for categorical variables, and the median has no meaning in nominal variables since there is no order to data.

Q: What does a large spread tell you about data?

A: A large spread tells us that there is a wide variation within the dataset from the mean.

Q: Can you think of a situation where measures of central tendency might be redundant?

A: In rare instances, data has a uniform distribution, which means that all values are equally likely. A measure of central tendency is not particularly helpful in that case.

Q: 'There was a bi-modal age distribution of [humeral shaft fracture]' [4]. What did the authors mean by the term 'bi-modal'?

A: The statement means that the authors found two different peaks of age when the humeral fracture was more common (the third decade in men and the seventh decade in women).

Q: When would you consider IQR to be a better indicator of the measure of spread compared to the range?

A: Median and IQR are better measures of data spread when data are nonsymmetric due to outliers.

CHAPTER 4

Why Average and Range Is Not Always Enough
Standard Deviation and Standard Error

I am particularly concerned to determine the probability of causes and results […] and to investigate the laws according to which that probability approaches a limit in proportion to the repetition of events. **Pierre-Simon Laplace**

 Learning Outcomes

We shall discuss the following material in this chapter:
- The variance and its importance
- The standard deviation and how to calculate it
- Why do we need Bessel's correction
- The standard error of the mean and how we calculate it

Standard Deviation: A New Kind of Average

Let us consider our swimming buddies; we went back to meet them and found a different group; then we made a third visit and plotted the observations from the three trips in the table below (Table 4.1):

Gr 1	6	8	9	10	11	12	13
n=	1	1	1	3	2	1	1
Gr 2	7	9	10	11	13		
n=	1	2	4	2	1		
Gr 3	5	6	7	10	11	13	26
n=	2	1	2	3	1	1	1

Table 4.1 Age of swimmers.

While relaying information about the three different groups we met, we found that the measures of central tendency are identical. **Mean, median** and **mode** are all **10!** How do we differentiate *between* the groups?

Did You Know?

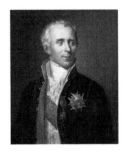

© James Posselwhite / Public domain [1].

Figure 4.1 Pierre - Simon Laplace(1749–1827), was a French polymath. Although mainly known for his contribution to physics and astronomy, Laplace also played an important role in advancing the discipline of statistics. He was the first to prove the Central Limit Theorem, a fundamental principle underpinning the law of probability in medical statistics [2].

Bullet Points

SD:

D stands for **D**ata **D**eviation

SD is affected by data deviation from the mean

Sample standard deviation is **S**

Population standard deviation is **σ**

When sample size is ≥ 60, the **sample SD (S)** is a reliable estimate of **population SD (σ)** [3].

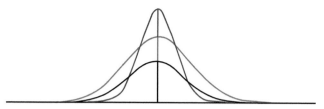

Figure 4.2 Plotting three different datasets with exactly the same mean, median and mode but variation in data spread.

Figure 4.2 shows three different datasets with identical measures of central tendency but different spreads plotted against each other. When we plot such data, the central line will overlap on each other due to the identical mean, median and mode values. The width of the curve will differ because of the variation in the spread of data. We could describe range and quartiles, but their usefulness in understanding variation is limited because variability is more than just range. We need a better measure of data spread. We do have a candidate, and it is known as the **standard deviation** (SD). SD is an *average* measure of the extent to which *individual data varies* from the *mean* (Figure 4.3).

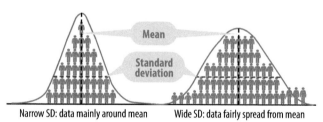

Narrow SD: data mainly around mean   Wide SD: data fairly spread from mean

Figure 4.3 Measuring heights, comparing data with narrow versus wide standard deviation.

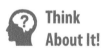

Think About It!

Should one always use mean and SD to describe numerical data?

A small SD means data are relatively close to the mean, and a large SD means data are more spread away from the mean, i.e. there is more variability in data compared to the mean value (most individuals are of average height in the left-hand figure, but there is a higher number of shorter and taller individuals in the right-hand figure).

How Do We Calculate Standard Deviation?

First of all, we need to calculate the mean value. Next, we calculate the individual differences from the mean, square the differences (Figure 4.4), then next we add the squared differences together and divide the sum by n-1, this is the sample **variance** (S^2). We need to square root the S^2 to find the **SD**.

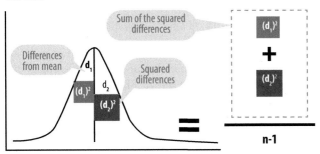

Figure 4.4 Calculating variance: sum of the squared differences divided by n-1.

Let's see an example. Looking back at our group of swimmers: the mean age of **group 1** swimmers is 10. The sum of squared differences from the mean (10) is 36, and this is divided by n-1 (9) to find the variance (S^2) = 4, the **SD** (S) is $\sqrt{4} = $ **2**.

Similarly, the variance (S^2) for **group 2** swimmers is 2.44, the **SD** (S) is $\sqrt{2.44} = $ **1.56**.

The variance for **group 3** is 35, the SD (S) is $\sqrt{35} = $ **5.91** (group 3, n = 11).

We now have a more precise idea of how the young swimmers' ages vary from the mean value.

A potential disadvantage of calculating variance is obvious if we look at group 3. There was a 26-year-old swimmer in that group. The age difference of this individual from the mean age is substantial. When the difference is squared, the difference becomes even more pronounced (variance of 35 versus that of 4 and 2.44). Squaring the value gives undue weight to extreme values.

Why Do We Use n-1 to Calculate Variance, Why Not n?

Since our sample is only a fraction of the actual population, any calculation made from the sample underestimates the population parameter. Changing the denominator to n-1

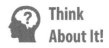

Think About It!

Why do we need to square the differences to find variance?

Is it always necessary to use the denominator n-1 to calculate variance?

What are the disadvantages of calculating variance?

Bullet Points

Sample variance: S^2

Population variance: σ^2

Sample standard deviation: S

Population standard deviation: σ

Variance: S^2

SD (S): $\sqrt{\text{variance}}$

S or S^2? They are just each other's alter-ego!

Bullet Points

When **mean** is described it is best practice to quote SD also to communicate the spread of data

For our **swimmers** the **mean age** would be written as such: mean age in years (SD),

Group 1: 10 (2)

Group 2: 10 (1.56)

Group 3: 10 (5.91)

Mean and (SD) are required for descriptive statistics

SE is affected by sample **size**

Mean and (SE) are required for inferential statistics

SE= SD ÷ √n

SE: is the **SD of the means**

helps to account for the underestimation and gives a better estimate. This rule is known as **Bessel's correction** [4].

Standard Deviation: A Better Measure of Data Spread

Mean and the **SD** complement each other when numerical data have symmetrical spread. **One** is a **point estimate** of the **centre**, the **other** of the **spread**. SD conveys information regarding the distribution of the values in the dataset around the mean value. When data are symmetrical, almost all of the data values distribute around 2 SD of the mean value. As we would find later, this principle helps us to detect outliers in the dataset and also proves useful for making probability predictions. SD can also be a guide to the precision of the sample mean. Let us see how.

The Standard Error of the Mean: How Precise Is Your Estimate?

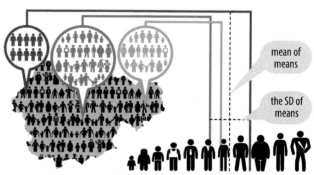

Figure 4.5 Calculating the SE of height (different colours represent different samples and their means).

We should be able to recall that the population mean is an unknown entity. We aim to estimate the population mean by calculating the sample mean. How do we know how accurate is our estimation of the unknown population mean? To appreciate this, we require another parameter, **Standard error of the mean (SEM)** or **SE** in short. SE is essentially the **SD of all the means** (Figure 4.5). SD is a measure of the variability of the data, and **SEM** or the SD of the means is a measure of the **variability** of the **means**. To calculate the SE, we need to take multiple samples from the same population and calculate their means and SD. Repeated sampling would have been rather demanding and is, fortunately, not required. Rather than taking multiple samples, we can calculate SE from our single sample with a quick formula (**SE = SD ÷√n**). **Calculating SE** from the sample gives us an **idea** about the **precision** of our **sample mean** compared to the **actual** population mean. A quick look at the formula would make it obvious that the *bigger* the sample size the *lesser* the error of estimation and the more likely the sample mean is nearer to the actual population mean.

Let's find out the SE for our swimmers: n = 10, √10 = 3.16; n = 11, √11 = 3.31

Group 1 SE = 2÷3.16 = 0.63
Group 2 SE = 1.56÷3.16 = 0.49
Group 3 SE = 5.91÷3.31 = 1.78

Placing Standard Error of the Mean in Context: The First Step to Inferential Statistics

We need to determine SE to calculate a range of values known as the **confidence interval (CI)**. The CI allows us to assess the range of probable values of the unknown population mean. Armed with the knowledge of the CI, we can begin to make inference regarding the larger and unknown population from our limited sample. If we wished to make inference about the likely age of swimmers from observing the first group of swimmers, we would calculate the 95% CI value of the swimmers' age to be:

Mean ± 1.96 × SE = 10 ± 1.96 × 0.63 = 10 ± 1.23

The numbers mean that we calculate it to be likely that the swimmers who come to this pool are between 9-11 (8.77 to 11.23) years old. *We shall learn more about CI later and why we use 1.96 in the calculation.*

We have learnt about measures of central tendency and spread; it is now time to explore sample distributions and what we mean by a symmetric distribution in the next chapter.

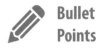

Bullet Points

SE:

how much variation we can expect in the means if we take multiple samples.

The **lower the SE** the **more likely** the calculated sample mean is **closer** to the actual **mean.**

SE is a measure of data pr**E**cision

SD is a measure of **D**ata variability

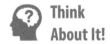

Think About It!

Why is SE smaller than the SD?

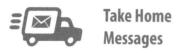

Take Home Messages

• Standard deviation (SD) is a measure of the variability of data. It is a better measure of data spread compared to the range.

• SD is the square root of the variance.

• We derive variance by calculating the individual differences of data values from the mean, squaring the differences, and then dividing the sum of the squared differences by n-1.

• The standard error of the mean (SE) is the standard deviation of the means of multiple samples from the same population.

• The SE is a measure of the precision of the data.

• The SE can be calculated from a single sample by the formula: $SE = SD \div \sqrt{n}$.

• The larger the sample, the smaller the SE.

• The smaller the SE, the nearer the calculated sample mean to the unknown population mean.

• SE is utilised to calculate confidence interval and make inference about the population from our limited sample.

Questions & Answers

Q: Should one always use mean and SD to describe numerical data?

A: No, these are superior measures of data variability but are only useful when data has a symmetrical distribution. When data are asymmetric in distribution median and IQR should preferentially be used to describe data.

Q: Why do we square the differences to find the variance, can the differences not merely be left as they are?

A: Since mean is the arithmetic average of data, the difference between a data point and the mean value will be negative for some values and positive for others. If we sum the differences, these differences will negate each other out, and the resulting sum will be zero. This is why we square the individual differences first before adding them up. Go back to the swimmers' age and check this out yourself!

Q: Is it always necessary to use the denominator n-1 to calculate variance?

A: n-1 is used as the denominator to account for the fact that sample sizes are usually small compared to the actual population. Therefore, if the sample size was large or included the whole population of interest, there will be no need to use n-1 as the denominator.

Q: What are the disadvantages of calculating the variance?

A: One apparent disadvantage is that variance is an artificial value and gives a large sum. Secondly, since the individual differences are squared, if there are extreme values, they contribute undue weight to the calculation of a variance. Finally, since variance is squared, the unit of calculation is different from the actual measurement.

Q: Why is SE smaller than the SD?

A: Standard error would always be smaller than the SD because the means of datasets will always be less spread out than the original dataset. Another way to look at it is the formula for SE= SD ÷√n. Hence, SE is always smaller than the SD.

CHAPTER 5

The Normal Distribution
What's So 'Normal' About It?

Whenever a large sample of chaotic elements are taken in hand and marshalled in the order of their magnitude, an unsuspected and most beautiful form of regularity proves to have been latent all along.
Sir Francis Galton

Did You Know?

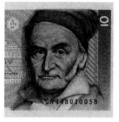

© Deutsche Bundesbank, Frankfurt am Main, Germany/ Public domain [1].

Learning Outcomes

We shall discuss the following material in this chapter:
• Data distribution and how to interpret it
• A normal distribution curve
• Explanation of a skewed distribution
• The z-score and how to calculate it
• The Standard normal Distribution
• The Central limit theorem

Figure 5.1 The normal distribution curve and its proponent **Carl Friedrich Gauss** (1777–1855), was featured in German ten Mark banknotes in 1989. He was a German mathematician and physicist who introduced the concept of Normal distribution [2]. It is also known as the 'Gaussian' distribution in his honour. He is rated as one of the most influential mathematicians of all time.

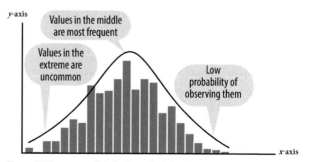

Figure 5.2 Frequency distribution of a dataset.

Let us start by discussing what we mean by data distribution. It is a display of the different values of a dataset. We illustrate data distribution by fitting a curve over a histogram.

By examining the curve, we can visualise how data are distributed in a sample (Figure 5.2). It is also known as a **frequency curve**.

The *x*-axis shows the value of **observation** and the *y*-axis the **probability**. The curve is a graphical probability plot of a variable. It is centred around the mean. The likelihood of finding *mid-range* values is *high*; the curve is **tall** in the **middle**. The probability of observing *high* or *low* values is *slim*; the **height** of the curve is **low** at the **two extremes**. The **total area** under the curve represents **100% of probabilities**. We can utilise this principle to calculate the exact probability of observing a variable of a given value. We can also make inferences from this calculation.

If the value of a given variable is observed at a *frequency* that is *at odds* with the calculated probability, that *variable*, and by extension, the sample, must belong to a *different* distribution. The distribution of random continuous variables, when plotted, assumes a *bell*-shaped curve (Figure 5.3). The curve is known as the **Normal** distribution. It is ubiquitous in scope and helpful to understand variation in our natural world, but that does not mean other frequency curves are abnormal! The shape of the curve is symmetrical, 50% of data are above and 50% situated below the mean. Most of the data cluster around the centre. The mean, median and mode values are all identical or nearly so and gather in the centre. The properties of the normal distribution are widely utilised in medical statistics to test for statistical significance.

Did You Know?

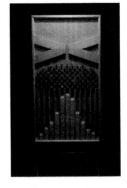

© Matemateca (IME/USP) reproduced CC-BY-SA 4.0 [3].

Figure 5.4 When beads are randomly dropped from the top of this machine, they gather below in a bell-shaped curve recreating the normal distribution. The board was invented by **Sir Francis Galton** [4].

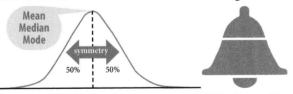

Figure 5.3 The bell-shaped curve compared against a bell, bit of a stretch but you get the idea!

How Do We Describe Normally Distributed Data?

We can describe symmetrically distributed data with the help of mean and the SD. The mean value (± 1SD) captures 68% of data, mean (± 2SD) encompasses 95% of data and mean (± 3SD) 99.7 of the data. This empirical rule is known as the **68–95–99.7 rule** (Figure 5.5).

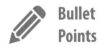 **Bullet Points**

The *total* area *under* the data distribution curve represents 100% of probabilities.

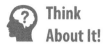

Think About It!

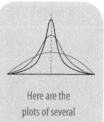

Here are the plots of several datasets, what is the distribution of these plots and what is the difference between them?

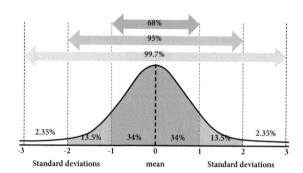

Figure 5.5 The 68–95–99.7 rule.

What Is Skewed Data?

Sometimes, we notice data distribution that is curved but not symmetrical, it has a long tail. The tail represents the **outlier**. An outlier is an extreme value on one side that pulls the data into a skewed appearance (Figure 5.6). The significance of a skewed distribution is that inferences that apply to normally distributed data are not valid for skewed data.

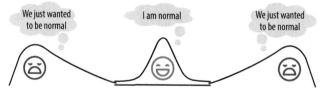

Figure 5.6 Normal versus skewed distribution.

What Happens to the Mean If There Is An Outlier?

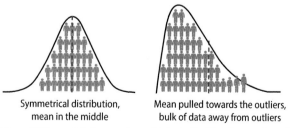

Symmetrical distribution, mean in the middle

Mean pulled towards the outliers, bulk of data away from outliers

Figure 5.7 Symmetrical versus skewed data, bulk of data is away from the tail in skewed data.

The measures of central tendency are variably affected by an outlier. *Mean* is *mostly* affected by the outlier and is displaced closest to the tail. Median is less affected. The mode value is not affected at all (Figure 5.7).

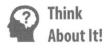

Think About It!

What Is Positive or Negative Skew?

A **positively skewed** data is one where the **outliers** in the data are **larger than the mean** value, and the tail is to the *right* of the curve (on the positive direction of the curve). Most of the values remain on the left. The outlier values unduly influence the mean value and displace it to the right of the median and the mode value. Median is a better measure of central tendency when data are skewed. Figure 5.7 above is an example of a positively skewed dataset. The converse is a negatively skewed dataset.

> Why is mode not at all affected by the outlier?

> Can mean and median values give us an idea about data distribution?

What Is the Point of the Normal Distribution?

Many numerical variables we measure are distributed normally, examples include age, height, weight, blood pressure etc. Understanding this phenomenon allows us to appreciate how individual data values are distributed within a larger dataset. The statistical tests we perform are dependent on the behaviour of the values within a distribution. If the dataset follows the normal distribution, we can employ these tests. Understanding this allows us to make statistical inferences from a limited sample. We can perform **parametric** tests when numerical data are **normally** distributed. If this is **not** the case, we perform **non-parametric** tests.

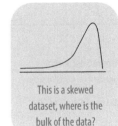

> This is a skewed dataset, where is the bulk of the data?

What Should We Do If Data Are Not Normal?

When data are not normally distributed, we perform non-parametric tests. These tests have the advantage that they do not require the assumption that data are normal. Parametric tests can tolerate minor deviations of data from the normal distribution. They are often *preferred* by researchers as significance tests since they can detect a *smaller* difference compared to a non-parametric test. *We shall learn more about these tests in Chapter 10.*

Bullet Points

Continuous **discrete** variables have a **Poisson** distribution, for example, *Independent* random events occurring within a time interval.

Statistical tests are used to assess data distribution but can be flawed, especially in too small or large samples.

It may be preferable to look at a histogram to assess the data distribution.

Converting a normal distribution curve to a standard normal one:

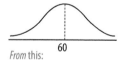

From this: 60

Figure 5.9a Normal distribution of exam score.

Mean of 60, SD of 10

To this:

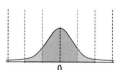

Figure 5.9b The Standard normal distribution.

Mean of 0, SD of 1

The *z*-score standardises the position of a **raw** score above or below the mean value by the SD.

Before we can perform a parametric test on a non-normally distributed data, first we need to **transform** it. There are various options for data transformation, **square or logarithmic** transformation being two of them. Data transformation can reduce the magnitude of data discrepancy and gives the distribution a more symmetrical appearance. For ease of understanding, the results of the transformed data need to be transformed back.

Here is an example of positively skewed data that was log-transformed (Figure 5.8). The new dataset is now suitable for performing parametric tests. Please note the difference in the mean value between the two histograms. The mean value of the log-transformed data will need to be anti-logged into a *geometric mean* to make it meaningful. The new geometric mean will not be identical to the arithmetic mean.

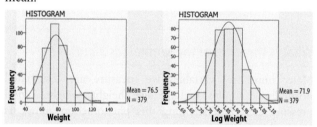

Figure 5.8 Skewed data on the left and transformed data on the right.

The Standard Score or *Z*-Score

Often, we have different samples in our hands with different scores. Previously we learnt that the standard deviation (SD) is an average estimation of the extent to which various datapoints deviate away from the mean. We also know that quite a lot of variables follow a normal distribution.

We can utilise these principles to assess the relative position of raw values compared to the rest of the dataset and make comparisons between different samples. First, we need to '**standardise**' each raw value by converting it into a standard score or *z*-**score**. Once the scores are standardised, scores from different samples can be compared.

Every sample will have its own unique mean and SD. To standardise them we first **convert** the raw sample into a **Standard normal distribution** (SND) so that the *mean* becomes a *universal* 0 and the *SD* is 1. Hence every sample will have a mean of 0 and SD of 1, and the scores will be comparable. Thus, we can compare the relative position of raw scores by identifying how many SD above or below the mean value the particular score lies: this is the *z*-**score**.

One example of the use of *z*-scores is our professional examinations. Suppose your **exam** score is **80**, the **mean** value is **60**, and the **SD** is **10**. Therefore, the corresponding *z*-**score** for your raw score is $z = (80-60) \div 10 = 2$, your score is **2 SD** above the mean. Congratulations for a stellar result! How do we put the score into context? We need to look at tables that give tabulated values for probabilities above or below the *z*-score. One can find these tables in many statistics books [5]. A *z*-score of 2 means 0.9744, or 97.44% scores below your score and 2.56% scores above (Figure 5.10). A *z*-score is useful to put into context population values i.e. height, BMI. weight etc.

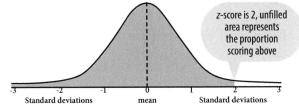

Figure 5.10 Interpreting the value of the z-score.

The Magic of the Central Limit Theorem

When we take a sample, we do not know the underlying population distribution. *Central limit theorem* dictates that **whatever** the **distribution** of the **population**, the distribution of the **means** will follow a **Normal distribution**. If we take lots of means from any distribution and plot them, the plot will follow a Normal distribution. We can utilise this fundamental principle to build confidence intervals and perform any statistical tests that utilise the mean value since we know exactly how the mean should behave.

We shall discuss in the next chapter how to estimate a range with a lower and upper limit within which it is likely the actual population mean will be found: the Confidence interval.

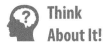

Think About It!

Why does a curve with wide variability have a lower peak than a curve with less variability?

Can you think of examples where we might come across a Poisson distribution in our working practice?

Bullet Points

Central limit theorem: it does not matter what the underlying population distribution is, the means of samples when plotted will display a normal distribution.

This is the basis for **tests** of statistical **significance** involving the **mean value.**

Only **caveat** for the central limit theorem is that for this principle to be valid the **sample size** should at least be 30 [6].

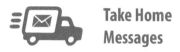

Take Home Messages

• Data distribution is a curve showing the probability of distribution of the values of a variable.

• The Normal distribution assumes a bell-shaped curve. Data are symmetrically and equally distributed around both sides of the mean in this curve.

• Outliers on one side of data distribution (too large or too small) will make the data distribution asymmetric.

• Asymmetric data distribution is known as a skewed distribution.

• Skewed data have a long tail.

• Positively skewed data have a long tail to the right of the mean value and vice versa.

• The mean value is displaced towards the outlier in a skewed distribution.

• We can perform a parametric test when the data distribution is normal.

• When data distribution is skewed, we either have to transform data or perform a non-parametric test.

• Any sample that follows the normal distribution can be converted into the Standard normal distribution with a mean value of 0 and a Standard Deviation of 1.

• Converting a sample into the Standard normal distribution allows us to calculate the z-score and compare z-scores between samples.

• The Central limit theorem states that the mean of samples drawn from any distribution with a sample size of at least 30 or more will have a normal distribution.

• Central limit theorem allows us to perform hypothesis tests involving the mean value.

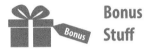

Bonus Stuff

More on the Z-Score

The formula for the z-score:

Z: the z-score, X: the raw score, μ: the population mean, σ: the population standard deviation

$$Z = \frac{X - \mu}{\sigma}$$

* the sample mean and the standard deviation is used in place of population values

Comparing Z-Scores

Table I. The age-matched BMD in ultra-distal and mid-distal sites of the contralateral radius in women with a Colles' fracture

			Ultra-distal*			Mid-distal*		
			z-score ≤ -2	z-score ≤ 0	z-score	z-score ≤ -2	z-score ≤ 0	z-score
Group	Number of patients	Mean age in years(± SD)	Number of patients (%)	Number of patients (%)	Mean (± SD)	Number of patients (%)	Number of patients (%)	Mean (± SD)
1 (Full)	211	59.5 ± 15.7	31 (14.7)	180 (85.3)	-0.94 ± 1.03	87 (41.2)	176 (83.4)	-1.63 ± 1.76
2 (No early menopause)	160	58.4 ± 16.8	22 (13.8)	138 (86.3)	-0.99 ± 0.94	62 (38.8)	134 (83.8)	-1.58 ± 1.60
3 (Early menopause)	51	63.0 ± 11.3	7 (13.7)	40 (78.4)	-0.77 ± 1.25	23 (45.1)	40 (78.4)	-1.84 ± 2.20
4 (Premenopausal age < 45 years)	34	32.4 ± 6.9	8 (23.5)	33 (97.1)	-1.52 ± 0.81	10 (29.4)	27 (79.4)	-1.39 ± 1.58

*the z-score is the number of standard deviations by which the patient's result differs from the mean of the age-matched reference group

Table 5.1 Reproduced with permission and © of The British Editorial Society of Bone & Joint Surgery [7].

Table 5.1 Authors were interested in investigating the association between distal radial fractures and bone mineral density (BMD) in women. Here we note the z-score. In this context, the z-score compares the BMD of a patient to the mean BMD of a patient of similar age, sex and ethnicity. The z- score is the number of SD by which a score deviates from the mean. The first row of the 211 patients represents the whole cohort. We can see from the first row of column five that 85.3% of patients had a z-score ≤0. The score means that most of the patients with wrist fracture in this cohort had a BMD score that was less than the age-, sex-, ethnicity-matched mean BMD value at the ultra-distal radial site; 14.7% had z-score ≤−2 (column four, same row); 14.7% of patients had a z-score 2 SD below the mean BMD of age-, sex-, ethnicity-matched population.

Questions & Answers

Q: Concerning the figure in page 28 demonstrating the plots of several datasets, what is the distribution of the plots and what is the difference between them?

A: All the datasets displayed have a symmetrical bell-shaped curve and have a normal distribution. The difference between them is that some of the plots are steeper than the others. The plots with the steeper curves have a narrower SD, and more data are centred around the mean value. The plots with flatter curves have wider SD and data deviates more so from the mean.

Q: Concerning the figure in page 29 showing a skewed dataset, where is the bulk of data?

A: This dataset has a negative skew as the tail is to the left. The outliers are smaller in value than the mean value. The peak of data is on the right. The bulk of data is away from the tail on the right side.

Q: Why is the mode value not at all affected by the outlier?

A: Mode is the most common value; it does not matter how large the outlier value is the most common value will remain the same.

Q: Can mean and median values give us an idea about data distribution?

A: The mean and median values are identical or nearly so in symmetrically distributed data. The more skewed the data, the more the mean is displaced. If there is a large difference between the mean and the median value, this would indicate that there are large outliers that have affected the mean value.

Q: Can you think of examples where we might come across a Poisson distribution in our working practice?

A: Hospital live births per month, the number of patients presenting to the emergency department every day etc. are expected to follow the Poisson distribution.

Q: Why does a curve with wide variability have a lower peak than a curve with less variability?

A: Where there is high variability in a variable's value, the SD would be wider. Since the total area under the curve always represents 100% of probability, the curve will get flat and the peak will come down when SD is wider and vice versa.

CHAPTER 6

Confidence Interval
What Is Your Guesstimate?

This problem consists in determining what arithmetical operations should be performed on the observational data in order to obtain a result, to be called an estimate, which presumably does not differ very much from the true value of the numerical character.   **J Neyman**

 Learning Outcomes

We shall discuss the following material in this chapter:
- The confidence interval (CI)
- 95% CI and how it is calculated
- Confidence Interval as a measure of effect size and hypothesis test
- Why 100% CI is improbable

Did You Know?

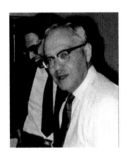

© CC BY-SA 2.0 de [1].

Figure 6.1 Jerzy Neyman (1894–1981), was born of a Polish father and a Ukrainian mother in current-day Moldova. A keen mathematician, his insight helped to strengthen some of the key concepts of modern statistics, including hypothesis testing and survey sampling. He introduced the concept of confidence interval [2].

How Confident Are You (With Your Guess)?

Invincible, strong or no clue? Wouldn't it be easier if we could quantify this in mathematical terms?

Let's Measure Heights

Let us assume that we are interested in the height of all employees of our hospital trust. It's a large employer with thousands of employees. We won't be able to measure everyone's height. We select and measure the height of 100 employees. We find that the mean height of male employees is 165cm and female employees is 150cm. We do **not know** the **actual mean height** of the employees of the trust but the mean value appears less than that of the average UK height. Are the employees on average short in stature? Let's take

Bullet Points

Confidence interval (CI): it reflects our uncertainty regarding the true but unknown population mean.

The *wider* the CI the *more uncertainty* there is.

95% CI is usually cited.

A working understanding of 95% CI is that there is a 0.95 probability that the calculated range contains the actual population mean.

CI is actually interpreted in the context of repeated sampling. *The correct interpretation is explained later.*

another sample. We choose another 100 employees, and this time, we find the mean male height to be 175cm and the mean female height to be 160 cm. Why this variation and which one is correct? What is going on?

They are both correct! We make guesses in life all the time. **Point estimates** gathered from a study are also in reality **guesstimates**. We say guesstimate because we *didn't* measure the height of *every single* employee. Instead, we chose a carefully *selected sample* and inferred the height of **all** employees from this **small sample**. Every time we choose a sample, purely by chance that sample varies to some extent from the actual population. This is the **sampling error**. We do not know how near **our estimate**, gathered from this particular sample, lies **compared** to the actual *true* population parameter. The study is an attempt at *guessing* the *unknown* parameter, albeit an educated guess. The bottom line is, we remain uncertain about the true value. A confidence interval is a measure of this uncertainty (Figure 6.2).

A confidence interval is just an uncertainty interval!

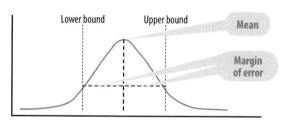

Figure 6.2 Mean and the range of confidence interval.

Think About It!

Would you describe 95% CI as a descriptive or inferential type of statistic?

Confidence interval represents a *range* of probable values within which we expect to find the true but unknown population mean. CI is a range with an upper and a lower limit that estimates the actual population parameter with varying degrees of certainty. There is always a trade-off in estimating the CI. If we wish to have a **narrower** estimate, the level of **confidence** in our estimate will be **less**, a **more confident** estimate will inevitably mean a **wider** margin and greater uncertainty. It is crucial to appreciate that **this is an estimate** and not a definitive result. Further, the actual mean could be anywhere in the illustrated example (Figure 6.3); the varying width of the red and green lines are due to the different levels of confidence. 95% CI (green arrow) is the most commonly used estimate, but this is not universal, sometimes 99% CI (red arrow) is also used.

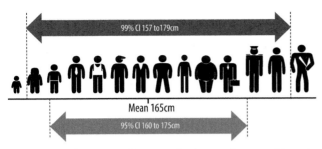

Figure 6.3 95% CI versus 99% CI, narrower but less certain versus wider and more certain CI.

How Is Confidence Interval Calculated?

We wished to estimate 95% CI of the height of all employees in an NHS trust. We started with a random sample and calculated a sample statistic. Next, we need to determine the sampling distribution of height. Height is a continuous variable and in a large sample can generally be assumed to be normally distributed. However, it is best to confirm this. For normally distributed data, the 95% CI for the sample statistic is:

Sample statistic ± 1.96 SE

SE is the standard error. 1.96 is the corresponding z-value for 95% CI. The calculation of the sample statistic $\pm$ 1.96 SE will, therefore, include the sample statistic with 95% of probability.

The advantage of CI is that it is a *range* compared to a single value of the mean and *better* reflects the *uncertainty* associated with calculating the unknown mean from a single sample. The width gives us additional information about the likely sample size and variability of the estimate. We get an idea about the likely range of results we would expect should we investigate the whole population.

Confidence interval is interpreted in the context of repeated sampling. The *correct* explanation of **95% CI** is that if we were to *randomly* take an *infinite* number of samples of the *same* size under *similar* conditions from the same population, and *repeated* the tests, **95% CI** generated from **95% of these samples** would contain the **unknown population** parameter. It is not clear which value within the CI is the unknown mean [3].

Bullet Points

What is 95% CI?

We do not know the actual population mean but we are 95% certain that the unknown population mean may be found anywhere within this range.

If the 95% CI of different means do not overlap each other, the difference between them is significant.

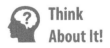

Think About It!

What is the significance of a z-value of 1.96?

Bullet Points

Confidence interval is not a point estimate but a range.

Confidence interval is useful to get an idea about the size of the effect.

95% CI can be interpreted as a significance test. If it does not contain the null value, the p-value will be <0.05.

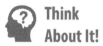

Think About It!

What is the implication of choosing 95% CI?

What is the problem of having too wide a CI?

Confidence Interval as a Hypothesis Test

We shall discuss conducting hypothesis tests in the next chapter, but it is relevant to briefly mention it here. We decide a test result is statistically significant when the p-value is <0.05. This threshold indicates whether or not there is a significant difference in outcome between the different groups. How big or small was this difference? We do not know. The p-value does not indicate it. A CI of the difference does. CI can also be used as a *significance test* similarly to the p-value. If the 95% CI of the *difference* between the two means *does not* contain the null value, the result is *significant* at a value of p<0.05 [4]. Here is an example. Authors were interested to investigate if statins reduced blood pressure (BP) in addition to cholesterol. Patients were given placebo or statin therapy in addition to antihypertensive treatment [5]:

> Pravastatin performed slightly worse than placebo, and between group differences did not exceed 1.9 (95% confidence interval −0.6 to 4.3mm Hg, p = 0.13).

The results would suggest that compared to placebo, statins reduced BP by 1.9 mm Hg on average, in the best-case scenario it may have reduced BP by up to 4.3 mm Hg. It may also have elevated BP by 0.6mm Hg. Since 95% CI of the difference in means crossed '0', the difference was not statistically significant. Statin was no better than placebo in reducing hypertension when given in addition to regular antihypertensives.

If the CI of the means of different interventions do not overlap each other they are significantly different. When they overlap they may still be significant [6]. Researchers compared the effectiveness of high-volume injection versus placebo in the management of chronic Achilles tendinopathy [7]. They assessed the primary outcome with the Victorian Institute of Sports Assessment-Achilles (VISA-A) questionnaire. The authors reported:

> The estimated mean VISA-A score improved significantly, from 40.4 (95% confidence interval 32.0 to 48.7) at baseline to 59.1 (50.4 to 67.8) at 24 weeks.

There was no overlap in the 95% CI scores at baseline and 24 weeks, we can conclude even without a p-value that the difference was significant (p<0.05).

Can We Be One Hundred Per Cent Certain?

We use the properties of the normal distribution to calculate the 95% CI. Since the possibilities in a normal distribution range up to infinity, it is not possible to include all the possible values of the true population statistic. Hence, we cannot construct a 100% CI but we can go pretty close, as close as 99.9%. Therefore, there is *always* the possibility that a CI constructed from a **single sample may not include** the **true population mean** (Figure 6.4).

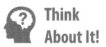

Think About It!

What is the probability that an estimate of the population mean based on the upper limit of 95% CI may be too small?

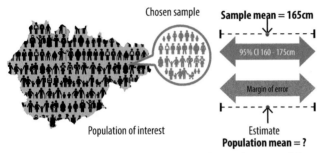

Figure 6.4 Best guess for the population mean is the sample mean and the margin of error, 95 times out of 100 the unknown population mean lies anywhere within the range of 160-175cm.

Since a normal distribution is required to calculate 95% CI of the mean can we calculate 95% CI for the median?

Let us review another research paper: authors were interested to assess if there was a sex difference in physician income and whether this was influenced by the sex composition of the practice [8]:

> The absolute adjusted sex difference in annual income was $36,604 (95% confidence interval $24,903 to $48,306) for practices with 50% or less of male physicians compared with $91,669 ($56,587 to $126,571) for practices with at least 90% of male physicians.

On average the sex difference in income was $36,604 (for the first group), but this could be as low as $24,903 or as high as $48,306. There was a sex difference in income that was more pronounced in practices with a higher proportion of male physicians. If the sample sizes were comparable, the variability between income was also wider in practices with a higher proportion of male physicians.

We are now perfectly poised to explore how to conduct hypothesis tests, but first, we need to understand the null hypothesis in the next chapter.

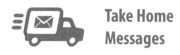

Take Home Messages

• The confidence interval (CI) is a measure of our uncertainty regarding the unknown population mean.

• CI is a range of values within which we predict, with a varying degree of confidence, the unknown population mean will be found.

• 95% CI is conventionally used in published papers, but 99% CI can also be used.

• 95% CI indicates that the unknown population mean may be outside of this range 5% of the time.

• The range of the CI gives us useful information about the size of the estimated effect.

• The range of CI can also be used as a hypothesis test of statistical significance.

• When comparing different interventions, if the CI of the mean difference between them does not include zero or the value of no difference, the difference will be significantly different.

• When we compare the effect of different interventions, if the CI of their respective means does not overlap each other then the difference between them is statistically significant. If the CI overlaps, the difference may still be significant.

• We can never calculate a 100% CI.

Questions & Answers

Q: Would you describe 95% CI as a descriptive or an inferential type of statistic?

A: 95% CI is an inferential type of statistic. We are estimating the actual population mean from our limited sample.

Q: What is the significance of a z-value of 1.96?

A: A z-value of 1.96 means the score is 1.96 SD away from the mean value on either side. The probability of a z-score more than 1.96 SD away from the mean value on either side is 2.5% or 5% for a two-sided hypothesis test.

Q: What is the implication of 95% CI?

A: There is a 1 in 20 chance that the true population mean will be outside this range. The constructed CI will not always correctly estimate the population mean.

Q: What is the problem of having too wide a CI?

A: A very wide CI demonstrates the impreciseness of our estimation of the unknown mean. The phrase 'not a clue' comes to mind!

Q: What is the probability that an estimate of the population mean based on the upper limit of 95% CI may be too small?

A: 95% CI means there is a 5% probability that the estimate may not contain the population mean. Since our estimates are almost always two-sided, there is a 2.5% probability that the upper limit may be too small.

Q: Since a normal distribution is required to calculate 95% CI of the mean can we calculate 95% CI for the median?

A: Yes, 95% CI can be calculated for the median as well as proportions, although the calculations are more complicated. A method known as Bootstrapping is utilised, for further details see Kirkwood and Sterne [9].

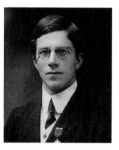

CHAPTER 7

Innocent Until Proven Guilty!
The Null Hypothesis

We may speak of this hypothesis as the 'null hypothesis' [...] the null hypothesis is never proved or established, but is possibly disproved, in the course of experimentation. **Sir Ronald Fisher**

Did You Know?

© Public domain [1].

Figure 7.1 Sir Ronald A. Fisher **FRS** (1890–1962), a British statistician, first proposed the null hypothesis. He came across the idea while devising a test to verify a claim from a lady. The lady claimed that she was able to detect whether milk was added before or after the tea was brewed by tasting a cup of tea: the case of **'the lady tasting tea'** [2].

Learning Outcomes

We shall discuss the following material in this chapter:
- The null hypothesis and the rationale behind it
- The alternative hypothesis
- How do we decide in favour or against the null hypothesis
- What is the test statistic
- How to calculate the p-value
- The significance of 'statistical significance'
- The difference between statistical and clinical significance
- What a p-value does not tell us

It is useful to visit the concept of universal justice to try and understand the **null hypothesis. Innocent until proven guilty** is the fundamental cornerstone of universal justice (Figure 7.2). Why do we insist on this even when it is obvious the accused is guilty? Because everyone has the **right to a just trial**, any presumption of guilt before the trial may unfairly affect the judgement.

The **null hypothesis** (H_0) is based on a similar principle (Figure 7.3). Suppose we are interested in testing the effectiveness of a treatment because we suspect the new treatment is likely to be better than the old one. However, when we compare the old treatment against the **new** one, it is similarly important to start with the presumption that the new treatment is **no better** than the **old** one.

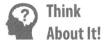

Think About It!

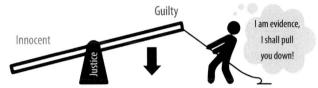

Figure 7.2 Universal justice, the default is innocent unless proven otherwise.

Let us assume Mrs. Ann Other has been charged with a crime, what is the null hypothesis and how will the case proceed?

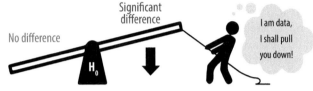

Figure 7.3 The null hypothesis, the default is no difference unless proven otherwise.

When the null hypothesis can not be disaproved, is it proved?

Thus, we ensure that unconsciously we are not biased against either treatment. Let us consider an example; suppose a new antihypertensive medication has been approved for use. After having used it in some patients, we wished to test if the new treatment might be a more potent antihypertensive compared to an existing medication. We decide to design a trial. Our **null hypothesis** would be **there is no difference in effect between the old and the new antihypertensive medication**. The hypothesis is mathematically expressed as $H_0: \mu O = \mu N$; if H_0 is correct any difference we notice between the means is due to chance and not a real difference. This is graphically illustrated in Figure 7.4.

Is it always necessary to have a null hypothesis of no difference in effect between the two interventions?

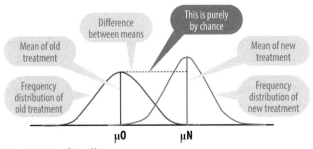

Figure 7.4 $H_0: \mu O = \mu N$

Legends to figure 7.4:

H_0 is the null hypothesis

μO is the population mean of the old drug

μN is the population mean of the new drug

Bullet Points

The trial and the statistical tests *both* tend to **favour** the **null hypothesis** unless data proves otherwise.

A **null hypothesis** is: a statement which we don't know if it is true, but we can only test if it is false.

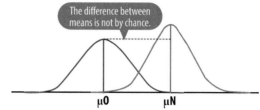

The difference between means is not by chance.

Figure 7.5 H$_a$: µO ≠ µN

We conduct the study, gather the data, and perform statistical tests. Our tests either successfully *disprove* the H$_0$ or *fail to disprove* it. If we **cannot disprove** H$_0$, we **can not reject it**. When we fail to reject H$_0$ we conclude that there is no difference in effect between the old and the new antihypertensive medication. Alternatively, if we can **disprove** H$_0$, we **reject** it in favour of the **alternative** hypothesis. The H$_a$ is: **there is a difference** in effect between the old and the new antihypertensive medication, the observed difference is real (Figure 7.5). **H$_a$: µO ≠ µN**

Therefore, the *hypothesis* test puts the *null* hypothesis on *trial*. Here is an example [3]. The authors wished to investigate if the presence of a full-thickness rotator cuff tear affected the clinical outcome in patients with proximal humeral fracture. They recorded several clinical outcome measures. The H$_0$ was:

There is no correlation between the presence or absence of cuff tear following fracture and clinical outcome.

On observing the results, the authors concluded:

The null hypothesis has not been disproved. There is no statistically significant difference in outcome with presence of an associated full-thickness rotator cuff tear with proximal humeral fractures.

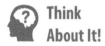

Think About It!

When the null hypothesis is rejected, which intervention does the alternative hypothesis support?

Note the authors **did not** write the **null hypothesis** has been **proved**. Instead, they employed a double negative. This is not just semantics. The H$_0$ is *never* proved. It is also easier to disprove than to prove H$_0$. Kirkwood and Sterne illustrate this point with an example; H$_0$: only non-smokers live >90 years. It is easier to disprove H$_0$ by finding a single smoker >90 years than to prove it by finding every single person >90 years and checking their smoking history [4].

The Test Statistic: Deciding For or Against the Null Hypothesis

Bullet Points

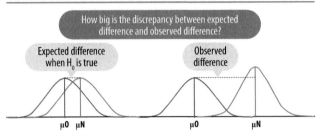

Figure 7.6 Calculating the test statistic.

Steps in a hypothesis test:

1. State H_0 and H_a

2. Choose p-level

3. Calculate the test statistic and p-value

4. Arrive at conclusion

We conduct tests to assess the null hypothesis. The test is known as a **hypothesis** or a **significance** test. It enables us to decide if the null hypothesis is false. When we conduct a hypothesis test first we calculate a value known as the test **statistic**. The test statistic is a calculation of the difference between our sample data and how it is expected to look if the H_0 were true (Figure 7.6). The test statistic will vary depending on the type of variable (categorical or numerical), the data distribution (normal or non-normal), the null hypothesis (superiority, non-inferior, equivalence) and the type of hypothesis tests performed (*t*-test, Chi-squared test etc). By calculating the degrees of freedom of a sample, we can place the test statistic in its correct position in the frequency curve. This will let us estimate the probability of observing a similar or larger difference for the observed sample size just by chance if H_0 were not false (Figure 7.7). This probability is termed the **p-value**. The test is nearly always two-tailed. By this, we mean that we are not sure if the effect of the new treatment could be better or worse than the existing one. We shall learn later that this means we would be prepared to reject H_0 if our test statistic fell on either side of the curve. *The full explanation is given later in the chapter.*

Research hypothesis may be based on prior observation that one intervention is **superior** to the other, but the **statistical hypothesis (H_0) is of no difference** (with rare exceptions).

Clinical equipoise: often there is genuine uncertainty about the effectiveness of an intervention compared to another. This is a position of clinical equipoise.

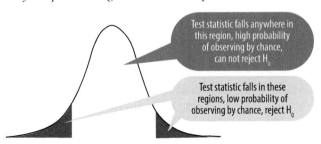

Figure 7.7 Placing the test statistic in the two-tailed frequency distribution.

Bullet Points

P<0.05 is the arbitrary risk threshold we are willing to accept to reject the null hypothesis, when it might actually be true.

Degrees of freedom: the number of values that can vary when the total value is fixed (for a sample size = n, it is **n-1**).

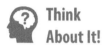

Think About It!

What is the implication of p = 0.05 threshold?

What is the probability of committing an error when p = 0.01?

What information do we get about the size of the treatment effect from the p-value?

What Is The Meaning of P-Value?

P stands for probability. **P-value** informs us what the **probability** is that in a hypothetical scenario where H_0 was true and there was no real difference between the means, we could observe a difference of the same or larger size by chance alone. Although we utilise a threshold p-value to decide for or against H_0, the **p-value** is better considered a *range* of probability *against* H_0. The **smaller** the **p-value,** the **greater** the evidence **against** the **null hypothesis** and vice versa (Figure 7.8). We learnt that before we can derive the p-value we need to calculate the degrees of freedom. This allows us to calculate the probability of observing the test statistic just by chance for the observed sample size.

Degrees of freedom (*df*) is n-1 (i.e. given a sample size, n = 251, the df is 250, if the test statistic was 18, we need to find the p-value for test statistic of 18, for 250 df). *A detailed explanation of **df** is given later.* Now that we understand the meaning of p-value let us choose a threshold for rejecting the null hypothesis.

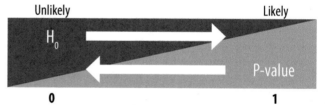

Figure 7.8 The smaller the p-value, the more unlikely the H_0 and vice versa.

When Do We Reject the Null Hypothesis?

We have learnt before that values in the middle of the frequency curve are most frequent and values near the two tails are very rare, these are the *rejection regions*. When we choose the p-value we set the threshold for the rejection region of the frequency curve just beyond the margin of critical value on either side of the frequency curve. Since our H_0 is mostly *two-sided,* if the test statistic falls in *either* of the two tails, we conclude that the result is *very rare* and unlikely to be due to luck or random variation. We **reject** H_0. If we find the **p-value is <0.05** this indicates there is <5% **probability** that we would find a *similar or larger* difference purely *by chance* if no such difference existed in reality. This is the critical value for rejecting H_0. Let's look at an example in Figure 7.9. If our test statistic falls nearer the mean value, the probability of it being observed is very high as this area has the highest peak. The test statistic marked by the diamond has a higher probability of being observed than the critical value. As we move further away from the middle, the probability becomes less frequent. When we find the triangular-shaped test statistic in the rejection region the probability of finding this value within the current distribution is less than the critical value. This is a rare outcome. So rare that we conclude this value is significantly different. A '*significantly different*' result has a **very low probability** of belonging to a **data distribution** that is **consistent with H_0**. We already learnt that our threshold for **rejecting** H_0 and concluding that treatments are **significantly different** is **p<0.05**. In that scenario, we are reasonably confident that this is not a fluke accident, but there remains a *1 in 20* chance we might have made a *mistake* and found a difference when there was none.

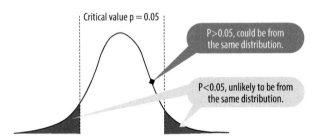

Figure 7.9 Choosing a critical value for rejecting the null hypothesis.

The Problem with Using an Arbitrary Threshold

The difference between p = 0.051 and p = 0.049 is not large. Yet, because of the arbitrary distinction of p<0.05, one result will be considered statistically significant and the other won't. In life, we rarely choose one or the other based on a difference of 0.2% (p = 0.051, 5.10% chance versus p = 0.049, 4.90% chance). It may hence be better to look at p-values as a continuum rather than a category: low p-values indicate that data point to strong evidence against the null hypothesis and high p-values indicate weak evidence against the null hypothesis [5]. Most journal editors now require absolute p-values to be presented and not written as 'significant' or 'not-significant'.

Bullet Points

We continue to believe that H_0 is true (i.e. the defendant is innocent) *until* evidence dictates otherwise.

P-value is our strength of evidence against the null hypothesis.

P-value: how likely it is that we could get a similar or more extreme result than the one observed just by chance if H_0 were not false.

A **hypothesis** test is also known as a *significance test* because when p<0.05 we interpret the result to be statistically **significant**.

Questions to ask *before* conducting a significance test:

- what type of data?

- how many groups?

- are the groups paired or independent?

- if numerical, are data normally distributed?

Types of test statistic

Significance test	Test statistic
t-test	*t*-statistic
ANOVA	*F*-statistic
χ^2 test	χ^2 statistic

Did You Know?

A lawsuit over a cold remedy forced the US Supreme Court to give a ruling on the relevance of statistical significance in March 2011 [8].

Matrixx, the manufacturer, was aware of reports that patients who took the remedy had complained of loss of smell, but did not pass it on to the investors.

When challenged in court the lawyers acting for Matrixx argued that the number of complaints were not statistically significant. Matrixx was under no obligation to relay them.

Unfortunately for the countless fans of p<0.05, statistical significance failed to win the day.

Clinical versus Statistical Significance

The **p-value** is an indicator of a **statistically significant difference** between the interventions. It gives us no information regarding the clinical implication of this difference. It is for the clinician to decide if the observed magnitude of difference is of any notable clinical benefit or **significance**. Let us consider another example; during the H1N1 influenza flu pandemic there was a rush to stockpile oseltamivir on the premise that it was effective against the flu virus. A subsequent systematic review noted [6]:

> In treatment trials on adults, oseltamivir reduced the time to first alleviation of symptoms by 16.8 hours (95% confidence interval 8.4 to 25.1 hours, P<0.001).

The p-value indicated that the treatment benefit was highly significant, but what about the margin of benefit, would you take this medication if it gave you as little as eight hours of symptom alleviation?

Clinically significant difference is a critical concept without which it is difficult to place statistically significant results in context. In another example, authors investigated if obesity affected clinical outcome after knee replacement surgery in comparison to non-obese participants [7]:

> Both groups achieved [*statistically*] significant improvement in outcome scores regardless of BMI, ten years postoperatively. All patients achieved the minimal clinically important difference (MCID) for OKS [*Oxford Knee Score*] and KSS [*Knee Society Score*].

The authors not only calculated the statistical significance of the change in outcome scores; they also noted whether the margin of improvement was clinically meaningful.

When to Perform What Type of Hypothesis Test?

We had a taster of hypothesis tests in this chapter. There are several of them and *we shall learn more about each test in the coming chapters.* Here is a helpful flow-chart to guide one choose the correct test (Figure 7.10).

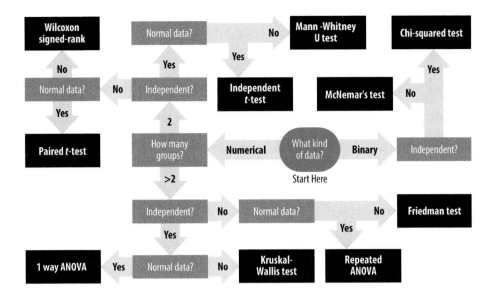

Figure 7.10 Flow-chart of hypothesis tests.

Why Is n-1 the Degrees of Freedom?

Many of us are familiar with the musical chair game. Figure 7.11 might help to explain why we use n-1 to denote the degrees of freedom. Suppose we had three players playing a modified musical chair. We have three chairs and all players get to choose one. The **first two** persons would be free to choose any chair they like, but the last person will have no choice. The **degrees of freedom** in this game is (n-1)=**2**.

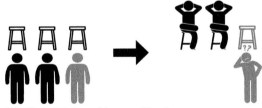

Figure 7.11 Musical chairs and degrees of freedom.

The process of accepting or rejecting the null hypothesis is not as straightforward as it seems. Let us see in the next chapter how mistakes can happen.

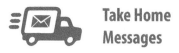

Take Home Messages

• The null hypothesis states that there is no difference between the two treatments.

• The alternative hypothesis states that there is a difference between the two treatments.

• The alternative hypothesis is two-sided and does not support one treatment over the other (one treatment could be better or worse than the other).

• The null hypothesis is a statement that we put under trial with the hypothesis test, usually at a significance level of $p<0.05$.

• We calculate the test statistic when we conduct the hypothesis test.

• The value of the test statistic is compared to the distribution of the test statistic to compute the p-value (for given degrees of freedom).

• If the p-value indicates that we cannot reject the null hypothesis, this means there is not enough evidence to disprove it.

• If we fail to reject the null hypothesis, that does not mean the null hypothesis is true.

• We have no proof that the null hypothesis is true; instead, it is not false.

• When the p-value indicates that there is strong evidence to reject the null hypothesis we reject it and accept the alternative hypothesis.

• When we accept a $p <0.05$, this means that there is a 1 in 20 chance we might have made a wrong decision and rejected the null hypothesis when it was not false.

• P-value only indicates if the observed difference is statistically significant. It does not indicate the clinical significance of the difference.

• The hypothesis test is also known as a significance test.

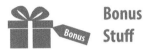

Bonus Stuff

How Any Margin of Difference Can Be Proven Statistically Significant with the Right Sample Size!

When we compare two treatments there is always a difference between them, however marginal. With a large enough sample size, it is possible to find a statistically significant difference for even the smallest difference. This does not mean the difference is of any meaningful value. When we conduct a hypothesis test, often the observed difference may not be large enough for the statistical test to conclude that they are significantly different. However, with the right sample size, the test can be fooled into thinking the difference is significant. Here is an example (Figure 7.12) [9]:

Table 1. Examples of results of significant testing using p value and comparative effect size

Example	Before	After	SD*	Diff.	n	t value	p value	Effect size	Characteristics
1	145	142	100	3	100	$=\dfrac{0.3}{\dfrac{3}{100/\sqrt{100}}}$	0.382	$=\dfrac{0.03}{\dfrac{3}{100}}$	Trivial effect & insignificant
2	145	142	100	3	10,000	$=\dfrac{3}{\dfrac{3}{100/\sqrt{10,000}}}$	0.001	$=\dfrac{0.03}{\dfrac{3}{100}}$	Trivial effect & significant

Figure 7.12 The same effect size but different p-value due to changing sample size.

© Restorative Dentistry and Endodontics, reproduced with permission.

* The t value indicates the test statistic.

Although the treatment difference is the same between examples 1 and 2, since the sample size is much larger in example 2 the difference in effect size that was deemed statistically insignificant in example 1 became statistically significant in example 2. Therefore, it is important to have the correct sample size in a study. We shall discuss the importance of appropriate sample size in the next chapter. The above example also illustrates why it is more useful to assess the difference in effect size and its clinical importance rather than to arbitrarily decide if two treatments are 'significantly different'.

Questions & Answers

Q: Let us assume Mrs Ann Other has been charged with a crime, what is the null hypothesis, and how will the case proceed?

A: The null hypothesis is, H_0: **Mrs Ann Other is innocent**, the H_a is, **Mrs Ann Other is not innocent**. The case will proceed with the prosecutor trying to prove beyond reasonable doubt that Mrs Ann Other is not innocent, there is no need to establish in the court that Mrs Ann Other is innocent. If she is exonerated it does not necessarily mean she is innocent, rather the standard for rejecting innocence was not met. The court failed to reject H_0.

Q: When the null hypothesis cannot be disproved, is it proved?

A: The null hypothesis can never be proved. If it is not disproved, we conclude that there was not enough evidence to disprove the null hypothesis. Since it was not disproved, we failed to reject it, but it is never proved. We never say the null hypothesis is true; rather, it was not proved false.

Q: Is it always necessary to have a null hypothesis of no difference in effect between the two interventions?

A: It is not always necessary. On occasions, a trial might be designed to test if the new intervention was not inferior to or equivalent to existing interventions.

Q: When the null hypothesis is rejected, which intervention does the alternative hypothesis support?

A: When the alternative hypothesis is two-sided it does not assume the superiority of one intervention over the other, only that they are different, it could be better or worse.

Q: What is the implication of p = 0.05 threshold?

A: There is a 1 in 20 chance that we might have rejected the null hypothesis by mistake.

Q: What is the probability of committing an error when p = 0.01?

A: P = 0.01 means the probability of getting the results by chance or committing an error is 1 in 100.

Q: What information do we get about the size of the treatment effect from the p-value?

A: The p-value gives no information about the size of the treatment effect. We need the CI to understand the effect size.

CHAPTER 8

Errors in Hypothesis Tests
Learn Your α From Your β

We must be able to reduce the chance of rejecting a true hypothesis to as low a value as desired; the test must be so devised that it will reject the hypothesis tested when it is likely to be false.

Neyman and Pearson

 Learning Outcomes

We shall discuss the following material in this chapter:
- Type I error
- Type II error
- The power of a study
- Factors that affect the power of a study
- Why prior sample size calculation is necessary before starting the trial

Did You Know?

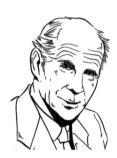

Figure 8.1 Egon S. Pearson CBE, FRS (1895–1980), was the son of Karl Pearson and a leading statistician in his own right. He succeeded his father to the chair of statistics at the University College of London and as the managing editor of the *Biometrika* journal. His collaboration with Zerzy Neyman led to the introduction of the concept of errors in hypothesis testing [1].

Type I versus Type II Error: False +ve versus False -ve

In the previous chapter, we discussed that errors might be committed when interpreting hypothesis tests. It may be easier to appreciate the different possible scenarios if we create a contingency table (Figure 8.2).

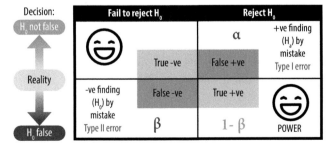

Figure 8.2 Type I versus type II error.

Bullet Points

Type I error: incorrectly rejecting H_0 (**false positive**).

Type II error: incorrectly failing to reject H_0 (**false negative**).

H_0: there is *no* fire

Type I error: no fire but alarm goes off

Type II error: fire but alarm does not go off

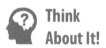

Think About It!

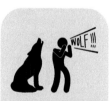

Remember the story of the shepherd boy who repeatedly cried wolf? You hear the boy cry out:

What is H_0?

In what scenario would you be committing a **type I error** and a **type II error**?

When the null hypothesis is **not disproved**, we **fail to reject it** (true negative), a truly negative finding; when the null hypothesis is **disproved**, we **reject it** (true positive), a truly positive finding; all is well and good.

When p<0.05, we accept a 5% risk that the null hypothesis might not be false, but we **falsely** reject H_0 and accept H_a. This is a **false positive error** since we are committing to a positive finding by mistake. It is known as the **type I error**. Conversely, there is also the probability that we accept the null hypothesis by mistake when it might be false. Thus, we **falsely** fail to reject H_0, thus committing a **false negative** or **type II error**. Let us consider a real-life scenario.

Fire, Alarm, Action

Many of us have lived as residents in hospital accommodation where the false fire alarm was not infrequent; toasters were a common culprit. A **false alarm** going off may be considered a **type I error**. Conversely, if the alarm battery was not maintained, a **fire** might **break out without the alarm** going off, this is analogous to a **type II error**.

Type I error: this is indicated by the Greek letter α

Type I error is entirely controlled by the researcher when the researcher chooses the risk level at which the null hypothesis is rejected (p-value). It is traditionally 0.05, but at times 0.01 level may also be selected.

Type II error: this is indicated by the Greek letter β

Type II error is related to several factors. One of the factors that is within the control of the researcher is the **power** of the study. Power is indicated by $1-\beta$.

The maximum acceptable limit of type II error is 20%. Therefore, the power of the study, or the ability to correctly make a true positive decision, would be 80%.

There is a trade-off between type I and type II error; the relationship is inverse. However, by increasing the size of the sample, one can lower the risk of type II error without increasing the risk of type I error.

May the Power Be with You

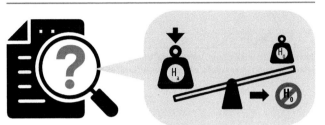

Figure 8.3 Power is the ability to reject H₀ correctly.

To understand power, let us deconstruct the following statement: **Power** is the **probability** to **correctly reject** H$_0$ (Figure 8.3). When we reject H$_0$, we accept H$_a$ (there is a statistically significant difference between the two treatments). If we are to **reject H$_0$ correctly**, the H$_a$ must be true. If we consider the distribution of the two treatments Rx a versus Rx b, if H$_0$ **is not false**, the distributions of Rx a and b will be part of the **same data distribution**, although not necessarily equal. The two **means** will **overlap a lot** (Figure 8.4a). Conversely, if H$_a$ **is true**, the distributions of the two **means will be spread** apart (Figure 8.4b).

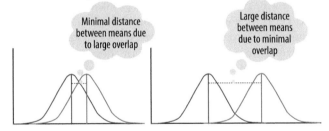

Figure 8.4a (left) H$_0$ true, large overlap between Rx a and Rx b.
Figure 8.4b (right) H$_a$ true, minimal overlap between Rx a and Rx b.

To detect the true difference between the two means correctly, we must be able to estimate them accurately. Let us recall here that the precision of estimation of means depends partly on the sample size. The smaller the sample, the larger the Standard error (SE), and the more imprecise the estimate of the population mean. Therefore, even if there was a real difference in the means, if our estimation of the two population means is inaccurate, there will be undue overlap between the estimated means. If the overlap due to the inaccuracy were large enough, even if H$_0$ was false, we may fail to reject it (Figure 8.5a).

Bullet Points

Power: ability to make the correct decision to reject the null hypothesis.

Power $= 1 - \beta$

Factors affecting sample size calculation:

Study power

Type I error

Standard deviation

MCID (Minimal clinically important difference)

Study design

Sample variability

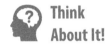

Think About It!

How can we reduce the risk of type II error in a trial?

What is the point of the power calculation?

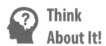

Think About It!

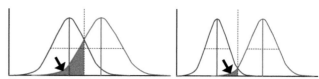

Figure 8.5a (left) Small sample, large overlap (large grey area, high type II error).
Figure 8.5b (right) Large sample, minimal overlap (small grey area, small type II error).

What does it mean to have a study with 80% power?

What Is the Power Calculation?

If we wish to avoid the situation illustrated in Figure 8.5a we need to undertake a power calculation. It is an estimate to identify the **minimum data** required to make a **correct decision** regarding the H_0, or an exercise to find out what is the **minimum sample size** we need to gather enough data to make the correct decision regarding H_0.

Can we design a study with 100% power?

As we increase the sample size, the precision of our estimated means will improve (Figure 8.5b). In this scenario, we can expect the estimated means to be a realistic reflection of the population means. If H_0 is false we shall have a high probability of rejecting it, we shall be able to correctly reject H_0, this is the power of the study: **the probability to correctly reject H_0**. If we come across a study that claims to find no significant difference between interventions, we must ask ourselves, have they had enough information to make **a good decision when it comes to H_0**? We have to satisfy ourselves that this was not a type II error.

Why do we need to perform sample size calculation, what about recruiting the largest possible sample size?

Is it enough to recruit a sample size according to the power calculation?

What Other Factors Affect the Power of a Study?

Several factors affect the power of a study. The sample size is the most important one, but other factors include:

- Type I error: inverse relation between type I and type II error

- Type II error: power is $1-\beta$

Would power calculation not be more precise if we performed it after we completed the study?

- Variability of data: the more variable the data, the less the power of a study

- Effect size: this is the smallest clinically meaningful

effect that would be of interest (MCID), it also has an inverse relation with power.

These parameters are all related to each other. When performing a sample size calculation, we need to consider all these factors (Figure 8.6).

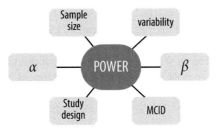

Figure 8.6 Factors affecting the power of a study.

How Do I Know What the Correct Sample Size Will Be When the Study Has Not Yet Started?

Sample size estimation is imprecise and only a guide. Often researchers would conduct a pilot study to identify the sample variability. We can fix type I error, and usually also have an idea about the MCID from pilot studies. If no pilot study was conducted, we might be able to get an indication of likely sample variability from previous studies or observational data. Let us see an example [2]:

> The power calculation was based on the change in mobility scale. Assuming that the outcome measure of mobility has a normal distribution and for a two-sided significance level of 0.05, in order to have 80% power to detect a significant difference of one point in the mobility scale then a total of 264 patients would be required using a standard difference (SD) [sic] of 2.9 taken from a previous study.

Authors designed a randomised controlled trial to compare the outcome between two different length nail designs for treating hip fracture. Their outcome of interest was the mobility scale. A single point difference in the mobility scale was the MCID. SD was calculated from a previous study.

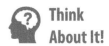

Think About It!

How can we tell if a study is too small if sample size calculations are not provided?

Which one is potentially more harmful, type I or type II error?

Bullet Points

MCID stands for minimal clinically important difference, the smallest clinically meaningful margin of difference.

If the therapeutic benefit of a drug is **statistically significant** but does **not reach the threshold of MCID,** the effect is not clinically beneficial.

Bullet Points

Sample size calculation is not precise.

It is the *best-case scenario* for required data (events).

Correct sample size is vital. A sample size too large or too small may result in incorrect conclusion concerning the null hypothesis.

Scrutinise Study Power When Results Are Non-Significant

We must scrutinise power when a study reports non-significant results. The abstract from the paper below illustrates this issue. The authors wished to demonstrate how small sample size and power might lead to misleading results. The SPRINT trial was a prospective trial assessing the outcome of reamed versus unreamed intramedullary nail in the management of patients with tibial fracture [3]. The primary outcome was re-operation. The authors analysed the primary outcome by comparing treatment groups at sample sizes of 50, 100, and in increments of 100 until the final sample size of 543. They commented:

> In the final analysis, there was a statistically significant decreased risk of re-operation with reamed nails for closed fractures (relative risk reduction 35%). Results for the first 35 patients enrolled suggested that reamed nails increased the risk of re-operation in closed fractures by 165%. Only after 543 patients with closed fractures were enrolled did the results reflect the final advantage for reamed nails in this subgroup.

The findings highlight the risks of conducting a trial with small sample size. Despite this, the prevalence of trials with suspicious non-significant results is widespread in medicine and is not limited to any speciality [4].

Is It Enough to Simply Report the Sample Size Calculation?

We have noted previously that sample size calculation requires consideration of many factors. It is not a simple arithmetic calculation. Therefore, it is best practice to cite clearly how these requirements were met. For example, what is the evidence of variability of data (SD), how do we know what the MCID is, etc.? There is evidence that reporting of sample size calculation in the medical literature is opaque and generally not satisfactory [5]. There are best practice reporting guidelines for this purpose: CONSORT (Consolidated Standards of Reporting Trials) [6].

Power calculation is crucial for planning a trial. Let's learn in the next chapter what are the other essential elements of designing a trial.

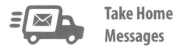

Take Home Messages

- When we conduct a hypothesis test and conclude on the statistical significance of the results, there are risks of committing errors.

- There are two types of errors: type I and type II.

- Risk of committing the errors is determined by the level of significance and the power of the study.

- Type I error is incorrectly rejecting a null hypothesis when it is not false; it is indicated by α.

- Type I error is the specified p-value (if p<0.05, it is 5%).

- Type II error is incorrectly not rejecting a null hypothesis when it is false; it is indicated by β.

- The maximum allowed margin of type II error is 20%.

- Risk of these errors is inversely related.

- Power is the ability to make the correct decision to reject the null hypothesis.

- Power of a study is indicated by 1- β.

- Power of a study should be a minimum of 80%.

- Increasing the sample size would increase the power of the study.

- A priori sample size calculation is essential to reduce the risk of type II error.

- Sample size should be carefully scrutinised in every study and especially where the study reports a finding of no significant difference.

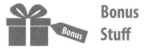

Bonus Stuff

The Type I and Type II Error, Power and the Critical Value

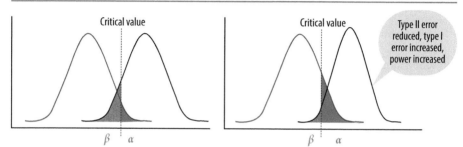

Figure 8.7 The relationship between type I and type II error illustrated (left), how the errors are inter-related (right).

It may be useful to have a graphical illustration of the relationship between type I and type II error. When we consider H_0 and H_a, they each have a frequency distribution. The margin of overlap between the H_0 distribution and H_a distribution depends on the mean difference. Let's suppose that the red curve is the frequency distribution if H_0 is true, and the black curve is the frequency distribution if H_a is true (Figure 8.7 left). All other things being equal, the location of the critical value is the other factor that affects type I and II errors. If we reduce type II error by moving the critical point, the likelihood for type I error increases and vice versa (Figure 8.7 right). Please also note that a reduction of type II error increases the power of the study (power of the study is 1- β: the area under the black curve to the right of the critical value).

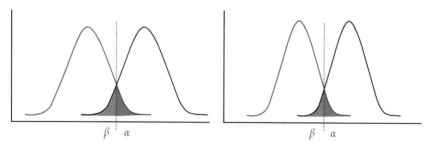

Figure 8.8 (left) Original sample wtih mean and variance, (right) new sample, n ↑, SE ↓, steeper curve.

In the figure above (Figure 8.8). We can see how an increase in sample size improves power. Increase in sample size results in narrower CI and less overlap between the two distributions. Even if the critical value remains at the same location, a smaller variance would result in a steeper bell-shaped curve with a smaller tail; the curves would move further away with less overlap; this would improve the power of the study.

Questions & Answers

Q: What is the null hypothesis concerning the story of the shepherd boy who cried wolf?

A: The null hypothesis is that there is no wolf.

Q: In what scenario would you be committing a type I error and a type II error?

A: We would be committing a type I error when we reject the null hypothesis and accept the shepherd boy's word that there are wolves when there are none. We would be committing a type II error when we accept the null hypothesis and ignore the boy's cry when there are wolves.

Q: How can we reduce the risk of type II error in a trial?

A: A simple option to reduce the risk of type II error is to increase the sample size and thereby increase the power of the study (power = 1-β). The conventional margin is to accept a type I error of 5% and a type II error of 20%.

Q: What is the point of the power calculation?

A: The point of the power calculation is to reduce the risk of failing to detect a real effect when it exists.

Q: What does it mean to have a study with 80% power?

A: The meaning of a study with 80% power is that provided the difference in effect exists in reality, if we repeat the study 100 times, we shall be able to find a statistically significant difference 80 times.

Q: Can we design a study with 100% power?

A: To get a study with 100% power, we would require a sample that has the whole population of interest.

Q: Why do we need to perform sample size calculation? What about recruiting the largest possible sample size?

A: It is unethical to have both too large or too small sample sizes. A sample too small would leave us open to the risk of type II error. A sample too large is wasteful of resources. Furthermore, if one of the interventions is beneficial, it is unethical to expose participants to the less helpful intervention or to deprive them of the beneficial one for longer than necessary.

Q: Is it enough to recruit a sample size according to the power calculation?

A: This depends on the design of the study. In prospective studies, one must account for likely loss to follow-up and increase the sample size accordingly. Otherwise, one may start with the required sample size, but as the trial proceeds, one may find that the study is no longer adequately powered.

Q: Would power calculation not be more precise if we performed it after we completed the study?

A: Power analyses should only be performed before we start a study. The mathematical and philosophical arguments required for a detailed answer are beyond the scope of this book.

Q: How can we tell if a study is too small if sample size calculations are not provided?

A: The required sample size is not merely a matter of a large enough sample, but it also depends on trial design, sample variability, MCID etc. When sample size calculations are not discussed, a useful indicator of the comparative sample size is the width of the 95% CI. If the CI is too wide, this would indicate excess variability in the estimation of the population mean. The study results were not a reasonable estimate of the actual population mean, and most likely, the study was too small for the requirement.

Q: Which error is potentially more harmful, type I or type II?

A: Considering that the accepted margin of type I error is 0.05 and type II error is 0.2, the figures indicate that researchers are less willing to tolerate a larger error in type I compared to type II error. This would indicate that type I error is potentially more harmful. However, it depends on whether you think it is a worse mistake to convict an innocent person (type I) or to free a guilty person (type II). The errors must be considered in the context of the null hypothesis, available alternatives, the seriousness of the condition, society's willingness to accept risk–benefit ratio and the cost-effectiveness etc.

If we are comparing a new treatment against a placebo agent and the H_0 is that they are the same, if we commit a type I error, we might be promoting a worthless drug to patients where there was no treatment anyway. Consider further the costs and the side-effects. If we commit a type II error and do not use the drug, we might deprive patients of a potentially useful drug. If we compare the new treatment against an existing potent treatment, if we commit a type I error, we might promote a drug that is no more useful than the existing drug. If we commit a type II error we deprive the patients of a potentially more useful drug, but an option is there. The choice is yours!

CHAPTER 9

The Randomised Controlled Trial
Why Does It Have To Be Random?

I shall here only observe, that the result of all my experiments was, that oranges and lemons were the most effectual remedies for this distemper at sea.   **James Lind**

 Learning Outcomes

We shall discuss the following material in this chapter:
- Why do we need to test treatments
- What is randomisation and why is it useful
- What is a confounding factor
- What is bias and examples of different types of bias
- What is the advantage of allocation schedule concealment
- Why is double-blinding useful
- What is a placebo effect
- Why patients can get better without treatment
- What are intention-to-treat and per-protocol analyses

Did You Know?

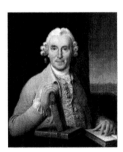

© Public domain [1].

Figure 9.1 James Lind (1716–1794), a Scottish physician, is credited to have conducted possibly the earliest comparative clinical trial. This led him to conclude that citrus fruits could protect against scurvy at a time when it was widely believed that scurvy was a disease of putrefaction. He published **A Treatise of the Scurvy** in 1753 [2].

When we propose to use a new treatment, we must first test it objectively against existing treatments. Why is this necessary? Because even if we propose new treatments with good intentions, they have **unproven beneficial effects** and can be **ineffective** or worse **harmful**. The medical literature is full of examples of untested new treatments that were used with good intentions but resulted in severe harm or even death [3].

When we compare two or more interventions against each other, the comparison must be done in an **unbiased and fair fashion** so that one arm of the trial is not unfavourably treated compared to the other. What are the pitfalls? It may

Bullet Points

Randomisation:
a method of participant allocation where the probability of allocation to either arm of the trial is dictated *solely* by chance.

When randomisation is *adequately* performed:

-the two groups may **not be identical** but **vary only due to chance**.

-the **confounding** factors are **equally** distributed.

be best if we illustrate this with a real-life example [4]. In this paper, researchers wished to assess if exercise therapy was superior to arthroscopic partial meniscectomy for knee function in middle-aged patients with degenerative meniscal tears. They started with clear inclusion and exclusion criteria. Participants who fulfilled these criteria were eligible for recruitment. Once patients were enrolled, the cohort consisted of a variable group of people with different demographics and co-morbidities. The researchers needed to ensure that patients in the two groups were as similar as possible so that we could safely attribute differences in clinical outcome to the treatment alone. To achieve this [4]:

> A statistician at Oslo University Hospital determined the computer-generated **randomisation** sequence.

What Is Random Allocation, and How Is It Useful?

Let's have a look at Figure 9.2; this is our population of interest. We want to test a new drug. We take a sample and divide the eligible participants into two groups to conduct a trial. Purely by chance, the two samples vary. We just learnt that for the result of the trial to be valid, the two groups must be as similar as possible so that the only difference between the groups is in the interventions received.

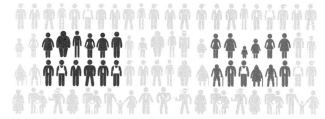

Figure 9.2 Sampling variation by chance.

Did You Know?

The trial of **streptomycin versus bed rest for pulmonary tuberculosis,** published in 1948 and run by the Medical Research Council, is arguably one of the first randomised controlled trials (RCTs) of the modern era [5].

Sample variation may unduly influence trial results. To ensure that the two groups are **as similar as possible**, we need to **allocate them at random**. Computerised programs are usually used to perform randomisation. We can also use random number tables. Date of birth, patient record number, day of the week, alternate patient etc. are not truly random. If we can distribute the cohort into **truly random groups**, the two groups will **differ only by chance** in demography, medical co-morbidities and other confounding factors.

What Is a Confounding Factor?

A confounding factor is a variable that is related to **both** the independent (treatment) and the dependent variable (outcome). In our previous study, exercise and surgery were the two independent variables and knee function was the dependent variable. Age in this scenario may be a confounding factor; relatively young patients might exercise more and have better knee function. If patients are not sufficiently comparable for age, it might influence the results. Some of these factors we know about, others we don't. The advantage of random allocation is that if we perform it appropriately, both known and unknown confounding factors should be equally distributed. Randomisation helps to **minimise allocation bias**.

What Is Bias?

Bias does *not* necessarily mean that researchers *willingly* prefer one or the other intervention, although this can happen. Bias is *any* systematic *error* in study design, methodology, analysis or reporting that results in *under-* or *over*-estimation of the effect of intervention so that we don't know the truth. Bias can affect the conduct of a study at every stage. Here, we are reviewing every stage of a study to learn how bias can affect it.

Allocation Schedule Concealment: Hiding Who Gets What

Once patients have been allocated to a trial arm, the schedule is kept hidden from the caregivers. This is known as **allocation schedule concealment**. It is done to prevent the caregivers from working out in advance the allocation of the next eligible participant. Lack of advance knowledge prevents them from preferentially allocating study participants to a trial arm. For example, recruiting unhealthier participants to the intervention arm of the trial in the belief that the participant is likely to benefit more from the treatment.

Bullet Points

Confounding factor: a variable that is related to both the independent and the dependent variables (Figure 9.3). It may or may not be measured.

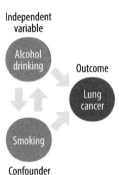

Figure 9.3 In the above example the increased prevalence of lung cancer in alcoholics might be due to them being concurrent smokers. This is a **confounding factor.** For the comparision to be fair there should be a comparable number of smokers in each group.

An **open-label trial** is one where participants are not blinded.

Bullet Points

Bias:
a *systematic* tendency to deviate from the true estimate of effect of treatment.

Random error:
non-consistent.

For a detailed description of the types of bias visit the Cochrane collaboration site [9].

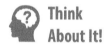

Think About It!

Do patients always get better due to placebo?

If clinical improvements are observed in a parallel-arm RCT that consists of a no-treatment arm, a placebo arm and a treatment arm, what is the margin of the true placebo effect and the true treatment effect?

Double-Blinding: Blind Leading the Blind!

Once participants are recruited, it is useful, if possible, to employ a **double-blind** technique where neither the participant nor the caregiver is aware of the treatment status of a trial participant. Double-blinding helps to avoid a scenario where both the caregiver and the participant may believe, exaggerate, or reinforce positive belief about treatment benefit and influence the results (**detection bias**). This is necessary because of evidence that therapeutic effect is systematically over-estimated in non-blinded trials [6]. Blinding may not always be possible in surgical trials, especially when compared to non-surgical treatment. In that case, researchers may opt to blind the assessor and the statistician, as was adopted in the above example to avoid **assessor bias** [4].

The Power of a Sugar Pill: The Placebo Effect

Placebo (Latin): *I shall please.* Often, we come across a **placebo-controlled trial**. Placebo is an inert chemical substance or physical intervention without any known therapeutic benefit or harm. Here is an example: authors wished to investigate whether an injection of platelet-rich plasma (PRP) improved outcome after acute Achilles tendon rupture [7]:

> Participants were randomised 1:1 to platelet-rich plasma (n = 114) or placebo (dry needle; n = 116) injection.

Platelet-rich plasma was the treatment arm, and placebo injection was the control arm. It has been common practice in trials of new drugs to have a control arm of a similar-looking placebo pill. Despite no known effects, patients taking the placebo pill do report clinical improvement [8]. In case you wonder, the sugar pill does not have any magic property. The detailed ethical and psychological discussion of the placebo effect is outside our remit. Suffice it to say that it is understood to occur because the patient expects to get better due to the intervention. Occasionally, administration of the placebo substance might result in adverse effect. This is known as the **Nocebo** effect and similar to the placebo effect might partly be due to patients' negative expectations.

The Margin of Therapeutic Benefit in Trials

Even without any treatment, a patient can get better. This is likely due to the natural course of the disease and also due to any lifestyle modification, patient expectation, belief, regression to the mean phenomenon (*explained later in the chapter*) etc. in combination. When patients get better due to a placebo agent, the observed benefit is a combination of the effect of no treatment as well as the actual **placebo effect**. Similarly, when a patient gets better in a treatment arm, the margin of benefit includes **therapeutic benefit** as well as the placebo effect and effect of no treatment [10]. Figure 9.4 demonstrates the differences in therapeutic benefit between no treatment, placebo arm and the active treatment arm.

Even if we design and conduct a trial well but are not careful while *analysing* the results, we could inadvertently introduce **bias**. Let us see how.

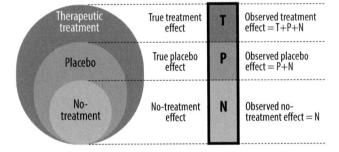

Figure 9.4 Outcomes in treatment, placebo and no-treatment groups.

Intention-to-Treat or Per-Protocol Analysis?

Looking back to our trial comparing exercise versus surgery for degenerative meniscal tear, the statistical analysis section reads [4]:

> All participants assigned to treatment were included in the intention-to-treat analysis.

What does it mean? Well, here is an extract from the flow-chart of patients recruited in the trial (Figure 9.5). It is evident that although the authors recruited seventy patients

Bullet Points

Options for statistical analyses in RCTs:

- intention-to-treat

- per-protocol

- as-treated

ITT is the gold standard in a pragmatic RCT.

ITT: 'Once randomised, always analysed'.

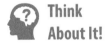

Think About It!

What are the disadvantages of ITT?

Apart from avoiding confounding factors can you think of any other advantages of ITT?

Of the three types of analyses which one has the most study power?

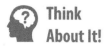

Think About It!

If there are a number of drop outs in a study, how would you wish to make up for missing data in ITT?

What is the best compromise between ITT and Per-protocol analyses?

Bullet Points

Intention-to-treat (ITT): a population-level effect.

ITT analyses the **effect of assignment** of a particular treatment.

Per-protocol analysis: analyses the **effect of adherence** to treatment assignment.

Regression to the mean: it is a natural phenomenon and may affect observation of recovery from illness or the effect of a treatment. If a random variable is extreme on the first measurement, it may regress towards the mean in the next and vice-versa.

to each arm, ten patients did not complete exercise therapy, and six patients did not have surgery. However, when the authors analysed the results, they treated all randomised patients as if belonging to their original allocated treatment group. Those **six patients** who **did not have surgery were treated as if they had surgery!**

That is precisely the case. ITT is a valuable strategy in a RCT [11]. ITT analyses **all** patients randomised in the trial in their original allocated group regardless of the actual treatment they received, whether they crossed-over to the other group or dropped out (Figure 9.6). There are arguments for and against ITT, but the benefits are apparent. If we fail to analyse patients according to their original allocation, we shall almost certainly lose the carefully achieved benefits of randomisation. The loss would introduce bias in the analysis due to the effects of confounding factors. A trial may be at risk of **attritional bias** when drop outs and losses to follow-up occur in a non-random fashion.

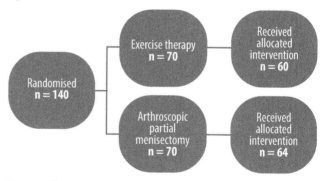

Figure 9.5 Flow-chart of treatment [4].

The alternative approach is **Per-protocol analysis** that excludes patients who do not comply with the trial protocol. A per-protocol analysis will only analyse those patients who **complied with the protocol** and, therefore, if there were substantial crossover, dropouts or loss to follow-up, the analysis would be biased. The illustration indicates the hazard of a per-protocol analysis, the groups would almost certainly be unmatched, and statistical analysis may not be valid. The third option is the **as-treated** analysis. Patients are analysed according to the treatment they received and not according to the original group allocation. As-treated analysis gives the maximum estimate of the treatment effects but is likely to be affected by bias.

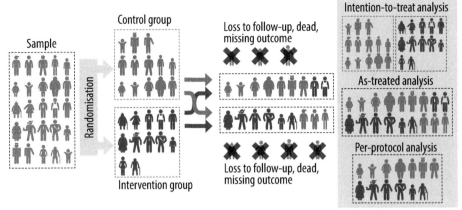

Figure 9.6 Options for outcome analysis in RCT.

Why Do Patients Get Better on Their Own?

Regression to the mean: random chance plays a large part in our everyday lives. A rookie footballer may do well in the first season but not so good in the season after. Everything regresses to the mean. Extreme events get diluted by average events which happen more commonly. It is essential to consider this phenomenon when attributing effects to an intervention. A disease will have natural fluctuation, patients may present to a physician when the symptoms are severe. Symptoms may improve without any treatment. If symptoms are measured when they are at the extreme, they are likely to be better when measured next. This natural fluctuation may give a misleading impression of patient recovery when, in reality, this was just due to natural variation.

Let us suppose we take a group of patients with a medical condition and give them a drug. We observe the outcome and conclude that medicine appears to have been highly effective. These patients might have improved purely because of the phenomenon of regression to the mean, not because the drug worked. That is why it is useful to have a similar group of control patients and compare the effects.

We have learnt about trial design, statistical analyses and the caveats thereof. Now it is time to turn our attention to performing statistical tests in the next chapter.

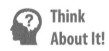

Think About It!

Between ITT and per-protocol analysis which analysis modifies the risk of type I and type II errors and how?

Can you think of a situation where ITT may not be the preferred method of analysis?

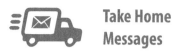 **Take Home Messages**

• We should fairly test every new treatment to avoid the risk of unintentional harm.

• A randomised controlled trial is the best design to test a new intervention fairly.

• Randomisation is a method of participant allocation where the probability of allocation to either arm of the study is dictated solely by chance.

• Randomisation is essential to distribute known and unknown confounding factors equally.

• Randomised groups are not equal but differ only due to chance variation.

• A confounding factor is a variable that is related to both the independent and the dependent variable and may affect the result of the trial.

• Bias is a systematic error that results in over- or under-estimation of one arm of the trial resulting in a deviation from the truth.

• Bias can affect a study in any stage: design, measurement, analysis or reporting etc.

• While planning a randomised trial, one must be careful to avoid several possible biases in selection, allocation, maintenance, measurement, detection, analysis, reporting etc.

• Participants in a trial can improve without any treatment for several reasons.

• Placebo is an inert chemical substance or physical intervention that when administered in a trial may result in detectable improvement in disease severity.

• Observed placebo effect includes both the effect of no treatment as well as the actual placebo effect.

• Intention-to-treat analysis is the gold standard in the analysis of randomised control trials.

• Intention-to-treat analysis is a pragmatic analysis and maintains the original allocation.

• Both per-protocol and as-treated analyses violate the randomisation of the original allocation and are likely to be adversely affected by confounding factors.

• While analysing results from trials, one must be aware of the chance variation of disease severity due to the phenomenon of regression to the mean.

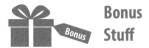

Bonus Stuff

Variation in Randomised Controlled Trials: Non-Inferiority Trial

An overwhelming majority of RCTs are designed to investigate the likely superiority of a new intervention. The null hypothesis, as well as the statistical tests, are designed accordingly. However, there is an alternative design of a non-inferiority type of RCT. Non-inferiority trials compare a new treatment against an existing treatment. Such trials aim to assess whether the *new treatment* is *not worse* than the current treatment. If it can be proven that the new treatment is non-inferior to existing treatment, we might prefer the new treatment for reasons of convenience, cost, application, availability, ease of use etc. In a non-inferiority trial, the **null** hypothesis is that the **new** treatment is **inferior** to the control treatment beyond an agreed clinically defined *non-inferiority margin*, it is a one-sided test (Figure 9.7). The **alternative** hypothesis is that the new treatment is **not inferior** to the control treatment, it could be the same or better. The p-value in a non-inferiority trial should be set at a one-sided value of 0.025 since only a one-sided test is being performed.

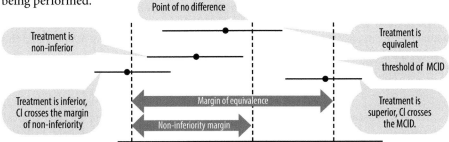

Figure 9.7 Difference between non-inferiority, equivalence and superiority trials.

Equivalence Trial

Equivalence trials are designed to investigate if a new intervention has similar therapeutic benefit to a control intervention. Both non-inferiority trial and equivalence trial designs are different to superiority trials, which assess if the new treatment performs better than the control intervention. The **null** hypothesis in an equivalence trial is that the **new** treatment is **not similar** in efficacy to the old treatment, i.e. superior or inferior. The **alternative** hypothesis is that the new and the old treatments have a **similar** therapeutic effect. An equivalence margin with an upper and lower margin is decided, and statistical analysis is performed based on the width of the confidence interval (CI). We *reject* the **null** hypothesis when we find that the *95% CI* of the margin of *difference* remains *within* the agreed equivalence margin (treatments are similar in efficacy). A difference may still be present between the two treatments, but this difference will not be clinically significant.

Questions & Answers

Q: Do patients always get better due to the placebo effect?

A: Patients do not always get better due to the placebo effect. In the same way that positive expectations may result in improved symptoms, negative expectations may result in an adverse outcome. This effect is known as the *nocebo* effect. For example, a recent study found that most of the side-effects of statins could be attributed to the nocebo effect [12]. Similar to the placebo effect, the nocebo effect may also be partly due to the worsening natural course of the disease. **Nocebo** is a Latin word and means 'I shall harm'. When a placebo agent demonstrates harmful effects, it is known as the nocebo agent.

Q: If clinical improvement is observed in a parallel-arm RCT that consists of a no-treatment arm, a placebo arm and a treatment arm, what is the margin of the true placebo effect and the true treatment effect?

A: The actual placebo effect is the difference between the observed total placebo effect in the placebo arm minus the effect observed in the no-treatment arm. Similarly, the actual treatment effect is the difference between the observed treatment effect and the combination of the placebo effect and the no-treatment effect.

Q: What is the disadvantage of ITT?

A: The disadvantage is that there is a potential for ITT analysis to include clinical heterogeneity, i.e. include a disparate group of patients, some patients had the intervention, others were in the control arm, some completed the study, others did not etc.

Q: Apart from avoiding confounding factors, can you think of any other advantage of ITT?

A: The other potential advantage of ITT is that it gives a likely estimate of the benefits of the intervention when used in clinical practice (some would refuse to take it, others stop taking it etc.).

Q: Of the three types of analyses which one has the most study power?

A: Intention-to-treat analysis has the largest sample size as the whole cohort is analysed. The alternative types of analyses, depending on the quality of the study, if there are significant numbers of non-compliance or dropout, may no longer have adequate power.

Q: If there are several dropouts in a study, how would you wish to make up for missing data in ITT?

A: There is no right solution to compensate for missing data. The best approach is to try and minimise dropouts or loss to follow-up. Several statistical approaches have been advocated, and the commonest one is to carry the value of the last observation forward. The gold standard is the multiple imputations method.

Q: What is the best compromise between ITT and Per-protocol analyses?

A: Intention-to-treat may underestimate the effect of the intervention but gives a realistic estimate of its likely practical effect. On the other hand, Per-protocol analysis potentially overestimates the effect of the treatment and may be affected by confounding. The best practice is to perform a sensitivity analysis by conducting both tests. Such an approach allows an assessment of the extent to which bias may have crept into the trial. Sensitivity analysis also allows us to assess the likely non-compliance rate of the treatment in practice.

Q: Between ITT and per-protocol analysis which one modifies the risk of type I and type II errors and how?

A: Due to the heterogeneity in the group, ITT analysis reduces the risk of type I error (false positive) and increases the risk of type II error (false negative). ITT analyses are likely to be conservative and are more likely to find no difference between interventions. Per-protocol analysis, due to loss of patients, may not be adequately powered and therefore likely to be at risk of type II error. Per-protocol analysis may also be at increased risk of type I error due to confounding since the groups may no longer be adequately randomised.

Q: Can you think of a situation where ITT may not be the preferred method of analysis?

A: As we have learnt before, ITT analysis may prefer non-inferiority. Traditional RCTs are designed as a superiority trial where ITT offers a conservative estimate of the benefits of intervention and may well be the preferred option. In a non-inferiority trial, this may not be advantageous as ITT is more likely to favour non-inferiority since any protocol violation may dilute the treatment difference between the treatment arms. In this situation, a per-protocol analysis may be preferred.

CHAPTER 10

Choosing a Statistical Test
To 't' or Not to 't'?

© Public domain [1].

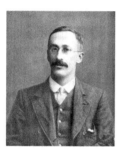

Did You Know?

> Now any series of experiments is only of value in so far as it enables us to form a judgement as to the statistical constants of the population to which the experiments belong. **W. S. Gosset**

 Learning Outcomes

We shall discuss the following material in this chapter:
• What type of significance tests to perform when comparing a continuous variable between two groups
• The difference between paired and independent groups
• The difference between the normal distribution and the t-distribution
• The t-statistic
• When to perform non-parametric tests
• The different types of non-parametric tests
• How non-parametric tests work

Figure 10.1 W. S. Gosset (1876–1937). Student's t-test was invented by an Englishman, William S. Gosset. Gosset published his paper in 1908 under the pseudonym *Student*. An Oxford-educated chemist, he was at the time employed at the Guinness brewery in Dublin. Company policy prevented him from publishing in his own name. He developed this test while trying to find a way to improve the quality of the company beer [2]!

We learnt previously about the different types of significance tests. The most common is the **t-test** which compares the difference of a continuous variable between two groups that are normally distributed. To calculate how different the two groups are we need a statistical parameter. The parameter for the t-test is the difference between the means of the two groups.

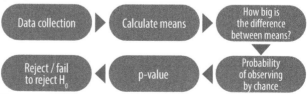

Figure 10.2 Steps in t-test.

Let's start with a practical example [3]. A researcher compared the haematocrit level in children with Tetralogy of Fallot (TF) between a control group with transferrin saturation >11.5 and a treatment group with saturation <11.5. The mean haematocrit level in the control group was 47.7 (range 35.2 to 58.2) and in the treatment group 60.8 (range 38.5 to 74.4). Is this a real difference or a chance finding? The author further commented:

> The t-test result showed significant differences [...] between the control group and the treatment group (p value<0.005).

Figure 10.2 shows the steps of the *t*-test. The test calculated a summary statistic, the *t*-statistic, which allowed the author to calculate the p-value. The p-value was <0.005, indicating strong evidence against H_0. This was real.

There are different types of *t*-tests. In the above example, the author compared the haematocrit level between two groups of participants. Data were **independent**. The two groups were **not related**. The **independent *t*-test** is the appropriate statistical test to perform when comparing a continuous variable between two independent groups (Figure 10.3). The H_0 for the above study will be: there is **no difference in haematocrit level** in TF patients with transferrin saturation above or below 11.5.

Bullet Points

Steps in the *t*-test:

- collect data

- calculate the means

- calculate the test statistic

- compare it to the *t*-distribution

- derive the p-value

The degrees of freedom:

Independent *t*-test:

$(n_1+n_2) - 2$

Paired *t*-test: $\dfrac{n}{2} - 1$

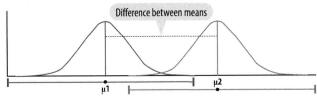

Figure 10.3 The H_0 of the independent *t*-test, there is no difference between the means; $H_0 : \mu 1 = \mu 2$.
H_a. There is a difference between the means; $H_a : \mu 1 \neq \mu 2$.

Contrary to what we have learnt so far, the **degrees of freedom** (*df*) for the independent *t*-test is not n-1; it is (n_1+n_2)-2. The alternative is the **paired *t*-test**. The treatment group had **repeated measurement** of haematocrit level following iron therapy. An independent *t*-test would no longer be valid in this scenario. The same group of patients repeatedly contributed data. The observations are paired. The appropriate test would be a paired *t*-test (Figure 10.4). The author further added:

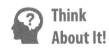

Think About It!

If Mr Gosset were testing the quality of two different batches of beer what type of *t*-test would he perform?

Bullet Points

t-test, also known as:

Independent samples t-test:

- Student's t-test

- Between-samples t-test

- Unpaired samples t-test

Paired samples t-test:

- Within-subjects t-test

- Repeated measures t-test

Paired t-test result showed significant changes in hematocrit levels before and after treatment (p-value <0.05).

Since observations are paired, we need a new H_0. The H_0 is that the mean of the paired differences in haematocrit level before and after treatment is 0. The difference between each pair is calculated and the mean of those differences tested against 0. The df of the paired t-test is $\underline{n}$ - 1 (n = total number of observations). $\quad 2$

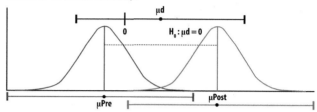

Figure 10.4 The H_0 of the paired t-test, $H_0 : \mu d = 0$, mean differences of the matched pairs is 0, $H_a : \mu d \neq 0$, the mean is $\neq 0$. (μd : the mean of the difference).

Parametric test assumptions:

- populations are normally distributed

- samples come from distributions with equal variances

What Do We Mean by a Parametric Test?

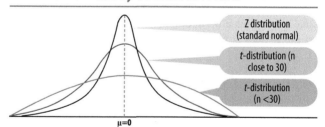

Figure 10.5 The shape of different distributions compared.

The t-test is known as a **parametric test**. The test is only valid when performed on normally distributed data. Continuous variables generally follow a normal distribution, especially when the sample size is ≥ 30 [4]. When sample **sizes are small, the normal distribution is not a good indicator** of data even if they are normally distributed. In this case, data follow the t-distribution. The **t-distribution** is not too dissimilar from the normal distribution, slightly shorter and fatter (Figure10.5). When the sample size is large, the t-distribution approximates the normal distribution. This is why we can perform the t-test for all samples of normal data.

What Is the Point of the *t*-Distribution?

The advantage of the *t*-distribution is that it takes the **sample size into account**. When the sample size is small, the *t*-distribution gives us a more prominent tail (wider confidence interval). The bigger tail accounts for the greater uncertainty in estimating the population mean from a small sample.

What Is the *t*-Statistic?

We have already learnt that when we undertake a statistical test at first we calculate the **test statistic**. The test statistic calculates how our sample data compares to the imaginary dataset if H_0 were not false. The test statistic for the *t*-test is known, rather imaginatively, as the *t*-statistic! The *t*-statistic is a ratio of the difference between the group means and the variability within the groups (Figure 10.6). It helps us to decide whether the observed difference between the two means is genuine or by chance alone. Merely subtracting the difference between means is not enough.

Bullet Points

t-statistic:
the ratio of between-group versus within- group variation in means.

Large *t*-statistic: groups are **different.**

Small *t*-statistic: groups are **similar.**

The **larger** the *t*-statistic, the **greater** the evidence **against** the **null hypothesis.**

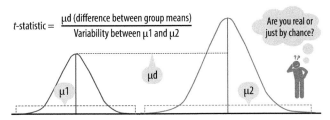

$$t\text{-statistic} = \frac{\mu d \text{ (difference between group means)}}{\text{Variability between } \mu1 \text{ and } \mu2}$$

Are you real or just by chance?

Figure 10.6 Calculating the *t*-statistic.

How Do We Calculate the P-Value from the *t*-Statistic?

We derive the p-value from the *t*-statistic and the degrees of freedom (df). *We have discussed df in Chapter 7.* It is the number of observations that can vary when the total value is fixed. We need to consult statistical tables to determine both one- and two-tailed (depending on the hypothesis) **critical values of the *t*-distribution** that is arranged according to different *df* and significance level. These tables are available in statistics books. When we use statistical software, it automatically calculates the p-value.

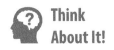

Think About It!

How will the variance affect our evidence against H_0?

Bullet Points

A *t*-statistic value of 2.5 means that the difference *between* the groups is **2.5** times *larger* compared to the difference within the groups.

We compare the *t*-statistic against the critical value of the **t-distribution** to derive the p-value.

If the **t-statistic** is **above** the critical value, we **reject H₀**.

What Do We Mean by the Critical Value of the *t*-Distribution?

Every test statistic follows a unique distribution. The *t*-statistic follows the *t*-distribution. The *critical value* of the **t-distribution** is the cut-off point at the junction between the non-rejection and the rejection regions on either side of the distribution. The cut-off point is determined by the pre-specified p-value (0.05 when H_0 is two-sided and 0.025 when it is one-sided), *for a review of the rejection regions please go back to Chapter 7.*

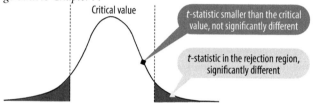

Critical value

t-statistic smaller than the critical value, not significantly different

t-statistic in the rejection region, significantly different

Figure 10.7 The *t*-statistic and the critical value for a two-tailed *t*-test.

Once we calculate the **t-statistic** of our sample, we **compare** it against the **critical value** to derive the probability (**p-value**) of obtaining a similar or larger value by chance. The test statistic will **fall** in the **rejection region** when it is **higher** than the **critical value**. A test statistic in the non-rejection region means that the value is reasonably common and the observed difference may well be due to chance variation. Hence, we *can not reject* H_0. A test statistic in the *rejection* region means that the observed difference between the means is *rare*, so rare that it likely comes from a different distribution than the one expected if H_0 were not false. We, therefore, conclude that the observed difference is very unlikely to be due to luck or random variation. It is **real**. We can **reject** H_0 (Figure 10.7).

Think About It!

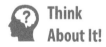

Why are the *df* different for *t*-tests compared to what we learnt previously?

The Mann–Whitney U test: Independent Samples

Let's see another example [5]: authors were interested in comparing bone health between adolescents with idiopathic scoliosis and a control group. They compared the bone health of 78 adolescents with idiopathic scoliosis with 52 age- and sex-matched healthy controls. There is no relation between the patients with and without scoliosis; data are independent. Therefore…

Analyses were performed with [...] the Mann-Whitney U test.

Although the *t*-test works reasonably well for data that do not strictly follow the normal distribution, if data are obviously not normal, a non-parametric test is the preferred option. The Mann–Whitney U test is the non-parametric equivalent of the independent samples *t*-test. We need a different parameter for this test. Instead of the mean difference, the Mann–Whitney U test compares the difference in ranks between the two groups. Apart from non-normally distributed continuous data, the test can also be performed for ordinal data. The H_0 of the Mann–Whitney U test is that there is no difference in ranks between the two groups, i.e. the populations are the same. The hypothesis is expressed as:

$$H_0: Rank_a = Rank_b, H_a = Rank_a \neq Rank_b$$

When we reject the H_0, we conclude that there is a significant difference in ranks between the groups.

If the two groups were entirely different, there will be no overlap in ranks and the groups will remain far apart. If the groups are similar, there will be overlap in ranking between them. The **test statistic, U,** indicates the degree of *overlap* **in ranks** between the two groups (Figure 10.8). The smaller the U, the less the overlap and the greater the difference between the two groups. To calculate the test statistic, we arrange all values in ascending order irrespective of the groups they belong to and rank them. If two samples are of unequal sizes a further calculation is performed after ranking to compensate for the differences in sample sizes. *A calculation of the U-statistic is demonstrated in the bonus section.*

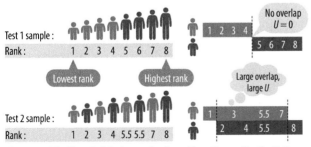

Figure 10.8 The U-statistic is the overlap in ranking; the smaller the U, the greater the difference between the groups.

Bullet Points

The non-parametric equivalent:

- independent samples: Mann–Whitney U test

- paired samples: Wilcoxon signed-rank test

Testing parameter:

Mean for parametric

Rank for non-parametric (values are assigned ranks)

Smaller *U*: bigger difference between groups

Contrast with ***t*-statistic, larger** the *t*, **bigger** the difference.

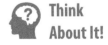
Think About It!

Why do we need a different hypothesis test for data that are not normally distributed?

Bullet Points

Non-parametric tests are free of distributional assumptions.

The non-parametric statistical tests do *not* directly compare the *median* value of the two groups.

The smallest value gets a rank of 1 and the largest value the rank of n (total number of values in both groups). We sum the ranks from each group and select the group with the smaller sum of ranks to calculate the U-statistic. A formula is available to make this calculation; it is cumbersome. Thankfully, modern software can perform it without any tears. The principle is to find out how many subjects in the group with the larger sum of ranks are smaller in rank than each subject from the group with the smaller sum of ranks. Next, we add these numbers together to generate the U-statistic. Finally, we need to satisfy ourselves that the U-value is **low enough** to indicate that the two groups are significantly different. We compare the U-statistic against the U- distribution table to obtain the p-value (Figure 10.9). We **reject H$_0$** if the U-**value** is equal to or *less* than the **critical value**.

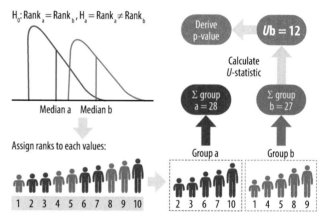

Figure 10.9 Steps in the Mann–Whitney U test.

Think About It!

Apart from distributional differences are there any other differences between the independent samples *t*-test and the Mann–Whitney U test?

Wilcoxon Matched-Pair Signed-Rank Test

The Wilcoxon signed-rank test is the non-parametric equivalent of the paired *t*-test. The H$_0$: **median of paired difference = 0; H$_a$: median of paired difference ≠ 0**. We compute the absolute differences between the matched groups and rank the differences (ignoring positive or negative differences) from the smallest to the largest in the same way as in the Mann–Whitney U test (Figure 10.10). Next, the ranks are signed (signed-ranks) according to their original negative or positive differences, turning them into positive and negative ranks. Finally, we add positive and negative ranks separately.

If H_0 **were true**, the **sum** of the **positive** and **negative ranks** would be nearly **equal** (larger and smaller differences cancel each other out, no difference between groups). The **test statistic** T is the **smaller** of the two sums. Is it extreme enough to have occurred unlikely by chance? We find the **critical value** by comparing the T-statistic for the number of pairs in the sample. If the T-statistic is equal to or smaller than the critical value, we reject H_0.

Bullet Points

Mann–Whitney U test, Wilcoxon signed-rank test: rank-based test.

Reject H_0 when U -statistics $\leq U$ critical

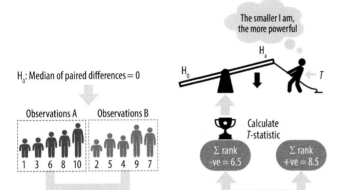

Reject H_0 when T- statistics $\leq T$ critical

Contrast with t-test: reject H_0, if t-statistics $> t$ critical

Observations A ranking	Observations B ranking	Absolute differences between pairs	Rank of the differences	(Sign)
1	2	-1	1.5	-
3	5	-2	3.5	-
6	4	+2	3.5	+
8	9	-1	1.5	-
10	7	+3	5	+

rank and (sign) of the difference

t-statistic is parametric

T-statistic is non-parametric

Figure 10.10 Steps in the Wilcoxon signed-rank test.

Please note that in calculating the T-statistic, when ranks are tied, they both get the average rank. If there is any value with zero difference this is omitted, **n** is the number of non-zero differences.

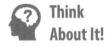

Think About It!

What is the disadvantage of a non-parametric test compared to a parametric test?

We just learnt what type of tests to perform when comparing two continuous variables, what if we had multiple samples? Let's review this in the next chapter.

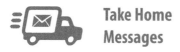

Take Home Messages

• The *t*-test compares the difference in means between two groups of variables that are continuous and normally distributed.

• The independent samples *t*-test is suitable for comparing two independent groups.

• The paired *t*-test is suitable where the same group contributes to repeat observations.

• The *t* distribution approximates the normal distribution when the sample size is large.

• The larger the *t*-statistic, the more different the two groups.

• The *t*-statistic is compared against the *t*-distribution to calculate the p-value.

• We reject the null hypothesis when the *t*-statistic is larger than the critical value.

• The *t*-test is a parametric test and requires distributional assumptions.

• Non-parametric tests are performed when the data distribution is not normal.

• Non-parametric tests assign ranks to data and compare ranks between two groups.

• The Mann–Whitney U test is the non-parametric equivalent of the independent samples *t*-test.

• The *U*-statistic is the overlap in ranking between the two groups. The smaller the value, the less the overlap and the more different the two groups.

• We reject the H_0 when we find that the *U*-statistic is equal to or lower than the critical value.

• The Wilcoxon matched-pair signed-rank test is the non-parametric equivalent of the paired samples *t*-test.

• The absolute differences between the paired groups are ranked, the ranks are signed and added together to calculate the sum of signed ranks.

• The *T*-statistic is the smaller of the two sums. The smaller the *T*-statistic, the lower the probability that the data arose by chance.

• If the *T*-statistic is equal to or smaller than the critical value, we reject H_0.

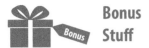

Bonus Stuff

Can We Test a Single Sample?

We have not discussed one-sample tests. The parametric equivalent is the **one-sample** **t-test**. The one-sample *t*-test compares the mean of a single group against a hypothetical mean. For example, if we wanted to test whether the height of our employees was significantly different from the national average, we could use the one-sample *t*-test. There are two non-parametric equivalent tests: the **Sign test** and the **Wilcoxon signed rank-sum test**. The sign test calculates whether the observations are above or below a hypothetical value. A better alternative is the Wilcoxon signed rank-sum test.

What Are the Other Assumptions Necessary for the *t*-Test to Be Valid?

For the *t*-test to be valid both groups need to be normally distributed and of similar size. Although there is no requirement for the two groups to be equal, comparing a large group against a small group is likely to give inaccurate results. The variances, or standard deviation (SD), of the two groups, should also be similar for the independent samples *t*-test. A rough guide is that the SD of one group should not be more than twice the size of the other. If the variances are unequal, this can affect the likelihood of a type I error. The SPSS package offers a Levene's test to check for the equality of variance and offers mathematical compensation to account for the difference. However, a better option may be to employ logarithmic transformation to reduce extreme differences in data or to abandon a parametric test and perform a non-parametric one [6]. We should ideally perform a *t*-test on interval data. Interval data are continuous data where the unit of measurement remains the same (of equal intervals). Examples include height, weight, age, time, distance etc. Satisfaction or pain rating scores, although numeric, (1-100, for example) are not truly interval. However, parametric tests are often performed for such data and may still be valid as long as the data are normally distributed. For an independent *t*-test, the observations have to be independent, not influenced by each other. For a paired *t*-test, the differences within each pair need to be normally distributed.

Is There Any Way to Perform a Parametric Test if Data Are Not Normal?

The *t*-test does allow for a minor departure from the normal distribution. If data are only marginally skewed, a parametric test is still valid. However, a non-parametric test should be performed if data are grossly skewed. This is the preferred approach for most medical journals rather than to try and transform data. Another option is to transform skewed data to reduce extreme values. This may allow for parametric tests to be performed. Sometimes this approach is preferred because parametric tests are more powerful and therefore more likely to detect smaller differences than non-parametric tests in smaller samples. Bland and Altman recommend this approach as entirely valid [7]. The final option is to perform both parametric and non-parametric tests and accept the more conservative of the two results.

Are Non-Parametric Tests Entirely Assumption-Free?

Non-parametric tests are not entirely assumption-free. The test assumes that data are rankable. The Mann-Whitney U test assumes no tied ranks. Mathematical corrections are necessary if there are many tied ranks [8]. The Wilcoxon matched-pair signed-rank test assumes that the differences between the pairs of observations are symmetrical. If this assumption is not met, the sign test is preferred by many [8].

The Calculation of the Mann-Whitney U Test

The calculation of the example in Figure 10.9 is reproduced below. When we compare the U- statistic against the U-distribution, we do not use degrees of freedom. We use n_1 and n_2.

Observations	Ranks	Observations	Ranks	Group a ranks smaller than Group b ranks
Group a (n_1)		Group b (n_2)		Calculation of U
2	2	1	1	4 (2<4,5,8,9)
3	3	4	4	4 (3<4,5,8,9)
6	6	5	5	2 (6<8,9)
7	7	8	8	2 (7<8,9)
10	10	9	9	0 (10>1,4,5,8,9)
Σ of ranks	28	Σ of ranks	27	$U = 2+2+4+4 = 12$

$U_{statistic}$ 12, $n_1 = 5$, $n_2 = 5$

$U_{critical}$ (5,5) = 2 at 0.05 level

$U_{statistic} > U_{critical}$

can not reject H_0

Please note that the calculations of the Mann-Whitney U test may differ between books.

Questions & Answers

Q: If Mr Gosset were testing the quality of two different batches of beer, what type of *t*-test would he perform?

A: Two different batches of beer are not related, therefore the appropriate test would be an independent *t*-test.

Q: How will the variance affect our evidence against the null hypothesis?

A: Variance will affect the variability between the groups; the more the variance, the less the t-statistic, the less the evidence against the null hypothesis.

Q: Why are the *df* different for *t*-tests compared to what we learnt previously?

A: The *df* are the number of independent observations. In an independent samples *t*-test, we have two different samples; the *df* are n-1 for each sample $(n_1-1 + n_2-1 = n_1+n_2-2)$. As for the related samples *t*-test, although we have two different samples they are paired; therefore, the unit of analysis is the matched pair, the *df* are $\frac{n}{2}-1$ (n pair-1).

Q: Why do we need a different hypothesis test for data that are not normally distributed?

A: The *t*-test calculates differences in means, but the mean value is adversely affected by an outlier. The results of a *t*-test might also be adversely affected by an outlier and incorrectly indicate a spurious significance. A non-parametric test is less affected by an outlier. Therefore, non-parametric tests are preferred when the data distribution is not normal.

Q: Apart from distributional differences, are there any other differences between the independent samples *t*-test and the Mann–Whitney U test?

A: The independent samples *t*-test looks for differences in the mean $(H_0: \mu_a = \mu_b)$, but the Mann–Whitney U test looks for differences in rank. Mean is a measure of central tendency; rank is not. The tests not only have different distributional requirements, they also test different hypotheses.

Q: What is the disadvantage of a non-parametric test compared to a parametric test?

A: When we conduct a non-parametric test, we convert the actual numbers into ranks. Continuous data becomes ordinal. In the process, we lose data variation. This loss makes a non-parametric test less powerful to detect a small difference compared to a parametric test and more likely to commit a type II error.

CHAPTER 11

Finding the Odd One Out
The ANOVA Test

Did You Know?

Among innumerable footsteps of divine providence to be found in the works of nature, there is a very remarkable one to be observed in the exact balance that is maintained, between the numbers of men and women. **John Arbuthnot**

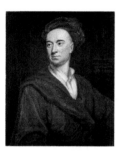

© Public domain [1].

Figure 11.1 John Arbuthnot FRS (1667–1735), a Scottish polymath, is credited with publishing one of the earliest works on significance tests in his work, ***An argument for divine providence.*** He consulted London birth records for 82 consecutive years to determine the sex ratio at birth. Having found a constant sex ratio, he concluded that the frequencies were too rare to have occurred by chance alone, it must, therefore, be, 'that it is Art, not Chance, that governs' [2].

 Learning Outcomes

We shall discuss the following material in this chapter:
• The appropriate significance test for more than two groups
• How does the ANOVA test work
• The different types of ANOVA test
• Difference between 'one-way' and 'two-way' ANOVA tests
• What is a 'factor'

The ANOVA Test

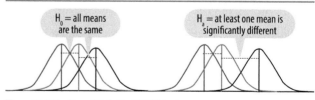

Figure 11.2 The H_0 and H_a in the ANOVA test.

In the previous chapter, we learnt how to conduct *significance* tests for **two** groups involving a *continuous* variable. There will be situations when we wish to compare **three or more groups** or more than a single variable. The *t*-test or its non-parametric equivalents would no longer be valid in this scenario. We need a different type of test for our null hypothesis. The **parametric** equivalent is the ANOVA (**A**nalysis **O**f **V**ariance) test. The **null hypothesis** of this test is that there is **no difference in mean scores** between the different groups. H_0 **is rejected if at least one of the means** is found to be **sufficiently different** from the rest beyond chance alone (Figure 11.2).

How Does the ANOVA Test Work?

All means may not be equal but if they come from the same distribution the H_0 would be true. We want to see if there is **at least one**, or more means, too far apart to be from the **same** population. The test statistic of the ANOVA test is the F-statistic. It compares the **variance between the groups** against that within the groups. If the variance within the groups is larger compared to the variance between the groups, then sample means are likely from the same population (Figure 11.3a).

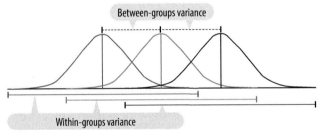

Figure 11.3a Between-groups variance < within- groups variance, F-statistic is small.

Conversely, if the between-groups variance is larger, sample means are unlikely to be from the same population (significantly different) (Figure 11.3b).

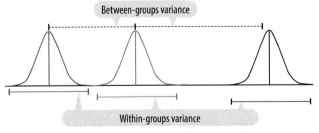

Figure 11.3b Between-groups variance > within-groups variance, one group is significantly different, the F-statistic is large.

Bullet Points

ANOVA is a **parametric** test. It requires distributional assumptions.

ANOVA: are all means part of the same population?

Compares differences in means between ≥3 groups.

H_0: $\mu 1 = \mu 2 = \mu 3$....

ANOVA versus t-test:

One-way ANOVA/ Independent measures ANOVA: akin to extension of the independent t-test.

Repeated measures ANOVA: akin to extension of the paired t- test.

Think About It!

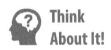

What is the drawback of a one-way ANOVA test?

Bullet Points

Variance:
it is also known as the **sum of squares.**

MSB:
mean sum of squares, between-groups.

MSW:
mean sum of squares, within-groups.

F-statistic:
the ratio of between- groups (MSB) and within-groups variance (MSW).

$$F = \frac{MSB}{MSW}$$

F is larger when the **between-groups** variance is **larger** than the within- groups variance.

Within-groups variation is also known as the **residual**.

How Do We Find the P-Value From the *F*-statistic?

We can not decide on the p-value based on the F-statistic alone (Figure 11.4). We also need to know the degrees of freedom (*df*). While conducting the ANOVA test we take into account two different *df* (n: total number of observations, c: total number of columns, our **between-groups df is c-1** and **within-groups df is n-c**). The **total *df* is n-1**. The tables in statistical books will specify a critical value of the *F*-distribution for the numerator df (c-1) and the denominator df (n-c). If our *F*-statistic is **larger** than the *F* **critical** value, we **reject** H$_0$ (Figure 11.4).

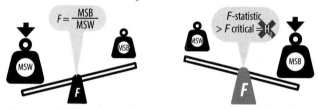

Figure 11.4 ANOVA: a test of variability ratio, small versus large *F*-statistic.

One-Way ANOVA

There are several types of ANOVA test. The simplest one is the **one-way ANOVA** test. If we wished to compare a single continuous variable between more than two groups, we would perform a one-way ANOVA test. Let us see an example. Authors wanted to investigate if prenatal nicotine exposure affected neurobehavioural development of infants. They compared neonatal behaviour between a group exposed to e-cigarettes, a group exposed to cigarettes and a control group not exposed to either. Neurobehaviour was compared between the three groups of infants. The **null hypothesis** was that there was **no significant difference** in neurobehaviour **between the three groups of infants** [3]. The **dependent variable** was neurobehavioural outcome (NBA). The authors commented:

> ANOVAs were conducted to assess group differences for [...] NBAs.

The results suggest that there was a significant difference between the three groups. The limitation of the one-way ANOVA test is that it only informs us whether there was a difference in means between the groups. The test does not identify which group was different. *We shall learn how to identify this later in the chapter.*

Repeated Measures ANOVA

If we take repeated measurements from the same participant, one-way ANOVA is no longer valid as participants contributed data more than once. We need a different test: **repeated measures ANOVA**. Let us see another example [4]. Authors wished to compare the difference of blood pressure reading measured between a routine clinic visit, in a quiet room and that using an automated pressure reading machine. The observations are related because the same participant contributed to the measurements using different instruments. The authors commented:

> We used analysis of variance (ANOVA; repeated measures if paired data) to reveal significant differences overall [...] ANOVA (repeated measures) showed a significant overall difference (p < 0.0001).

The results suggest that there was a significant difference in blood pressure between the three measurement techniques. Which one was higher?

Two-Way ANOVA

If we wished to explore two independent variables at the same time none of these tests would be valid, the appropriate test would be the **two-way ANOVA**. Authors were interested in investigating if there was a gait difference between laboratory mice trained with or without treadmill exercise and induced with experimental autoimmune encephalomyelitis (EAE) disease. The aim was to have a better understanding of Multiple Sclerosis (MS), which the EAE animal model closely approximates. Gait parameters were measured before the animals were experimentally induced. The **dependent** variable was the **gait parameter**. There were **two independent variables**, EAE disease and **treadmill** exercise. The **null hypothesis** for the **two-way ANOVA** has three separate components:

Think About It!

Why is ANOVA a better test than performing multiple *t*-tests?

What is the risk when we perform multiple *t*-tests?

Bullet Points

Factor: an independent variable in ANOVA test.

Two-way ANOVA: two independent variables.

$H_0 1$: no difference in means due to factor 1.

$H_0 2$: no difference in means due to factor 2.

$H_0 3$: *interaction* between factors 1 and 2 makes no difference to the dependent variable.

Bullet Points

The **Bonferroni correction** compensates for the increased risk of type I error when multiple hypotheses testing is performed by proportionately lowering the significance level. This is performed by dividing α by the number of tests (if 10 hypothesis tests are performed for α level of 0.05, the correction would amend the new α to 0.005) [6].

$H_0 1$: there is no difference in means due to treadmill,
$H_0 2$: there is no difference in means due to EAE disease,
$H_0 3$: the **interaction** of EAE disease and exercise does not influence gait (the independent factors do not affect each other's influence over the dependent variable).

The authors commented [5]:

All data were subject to a two-way analysis of variance (ANOVA) [...] the two-way ANOVA revealed an isolated effect of exercise ($p < 0.05$). However, there was a higher impact of the disease ($p < 0.0001$) and no interaction between exercise and EAE ($p > 0.05$).

The authors were able to reject both $H_0 1$ (exercise training significantly improved gait) and $H_0 2$ (EAE-induced mice had significantly worse gait). They were not able to reject $H_0 3$ (the interaction of exercise and EAE did not result in a significant difference in gait); exercise training did not improve gait in the EAE-induced mice.

How Do We Find Out Which Group Is Different?

The ANOVA test only informs us whether there is a significant difference between the group means, not which one is different. To find this, we need to undertake post-hoc tests without increasing the risk of committing type I error. There are several of them: Bonferroni correction (*see the side-bar*), Tukey's Honestly Significant Difference (HSD) test etc. Referring back to our initial study, the authors commented [3]:

Pairwise comparisons applying the Bonferroni correction for reflexes indicate significant differences between infants not exposed and exposed to cigarettes ($p = .001$) and e-cigarettes ($p = .002$). There were no significant differences found between cigarette exposed and e-cigarette exposed infants ($p = .236$).

The authors were able to conclude only after the post-hoc tests that there was a significant difference between nicotine exposure and no-exposure; the type of exposure (e-cigarette or cigarette) did not matter.

Let's see in the next chapter how to perform a significance test when the independent variables are categorical.

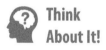

Think About It!

Do the means have to be equal for H_0 to be rejected in ANOVA?

Could there be a drawback to performing post-hoc tests?

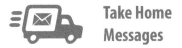

Take Home Messages

• The ANOVA test is performed when testing for significant difference of a continuous variable between three or more groups.

• The independent variable is known as a Factor.

• One-way ANOVA tests for the difference between three or more groups of a single independent continuous variable.

• Repeated measures ANOVA test is performed when the same group has contributed to repeated observations.

• A two-way ANOVA test is performed when we want to test the effect of two independent variables at the same time.

• The F-statistic compares the within-groups variance against the between-groups variance.

• The larger the F-statistic the stronger the evidence against the null hypothesis.

• The ANOVA test only informs us whether there is a difference between the means. It does not indicate which mean is different and to what extent.

• Post-hoc tests are performed for pairwise comparisons to identify which mean/s is/are significantly different.

• ANOVA is a parametric test that assumes that sample data come from a normal distribution.

• ANOVA also assumes equality of variance.

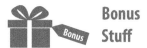

Bonus Stuff

How Do We Know How Different the Means Are?

This is calculated by the η^2 (eta square) value. η^2 is the proportion of variance accounted for by a factor. It is analogous to R^2 value found in linear regression. *We shall learn more about linear regression later in Chapter 13.* $\eta^2 = 0.01$ is small, $\eta^2 > 0.06$ indicates a medium effect, $\eta^2 > 0.14$ indicates a large effect. For example, the authors in the first study commented further [3]:

> Significant differences were observed across the nicotine groups for reflexes ($p<.001$, $\eta^2 = 0.338$), motor maturity, ($p = .002$, $\eta^2 = 0.145$).

The results suggest that although prenatal nicotine exposure significantly affected both neonatal reflex and motor maturity, the difference was larger for neonatal reflexes compared to motor maturity.

Are There Any Assumptions in ANOVA?

ANOVA is a parametric test. The samples should come from a normally distributed population, and the variances similar and equally distributed. ANOVA is robust to some degree of departure from normality. Each observation should be independent of other observations. It should be emphasised that when we test the assumption of normality, it is the residuals and not the actual data that are checked [7].

How Do I Know if Assumptions Are Met?

Distribution of data can be tested by plotting the residuals (the difference between the fitted and observed values) in a histogram. As long as this is nearly normal, the distributional assumption is met. Equality of variance can be tested by assessing the standard deviation or by performing the Levene's test.

What Should I Do if I Find that Data Distribution Is Not Normal?

When data distribution is not normal one can perform the non-parametric tests. The non-parametric equivalent of the one-way ANOVA test is the **Kruskal–Wallis test** and that of the repeated measures ANOVA is the **Friedman test**.

Questions & Answers

Q: What is the drawback of performing a one-way ANOVA test?

A: One-way ANOVA informs us whether the means between the three or more groups are significantly different. It does not inform us which one.

Q: Why is ANOVA a better test than performing multiple t-tests?

A: The number of t-tests required would increase with the number of groups in the test. This would be quite time-consuming. More importantly, if we perform more tests the probability of committing a type I error would proportionately increase. ANOVA has the advantage of performing multiple comparisons at the same time without increasing the risk of type I error.

Q: What is the risk when we perform multiple t-tests?

A: Let us see a mathematical example; we know that for a p-value of 0.05, each time we perform a hypothesis test we accept a 5% risk of committing a type I error. If we perform the same test thrice, our risk of error is: $(0.95 \times 0.95 \times 0.95 = 0.857$, our new alpha is 1-0.857) = 0.143. So, the overall type I error rate has increased to 14% from 5%. This is why multiple t-tests are to be avoided. If this is unavoidable, appropriate statistical compensations are required.

Q: Do the means have to be equal for H_0 to be rejected in ANOVA?

A: No, some difference between means is likely due to chance variation. We do not test for equality of means; we test if they come from the same distribution.

Q: Could there be a drawback to performing post-hoc tests?

A: Yes, post-hoc tests control for type I error by lowering the significance level, the risk of type II error concurrently increases, the power of the test becomes less. There is, therefore, a risk that small effect sizes might be missed due to comparatively lower study power. One way to avoid this drawback is to reduce the number of comparisons.

CHAPTER 12

Categorically Different?
The Chi-Squared Test

> On the criterion that a given system of deviations from the probable in the case of a correlated system of variables is such that it can be reasonably supposed to have arisen from random sampling.
>
> **Karl Pearson**

Did You Know?

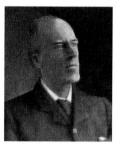

© Public domain [1].

Figure 12.1 Karl Pearson FRS (1857–1936), was an English mathematician who is considered to be the 'father' of modern statistics. He established the first university department of statistics at University College London in 1911. Karl Pearson developed the Chi-Squared test. The test is also known as Pearson's Chi-Squared test. He also developed the Pearson's correlation coefficient [2].

 Learning Outcomes

We shall discuss the following material in this chapter:
- When do we perform the Chi-Squared test
- How does the Chi-Squared test work
- What is the Chi-Squared statistic
- When do we reject the null hypothesis
- The types of Chi-Squared tests
- The null hypothesis of the Chi-Squared goodness of fit test
- The null hypothesis of the Chi-Squared test of association
- How to construct a contingency table

In the previous chapters, we learnt how to test our null hypothesis when the variable is a continuous one. When we collect categorical data, we group them into counts or frequencies. We need a different type of hypothesis test. Enter the **Chi-Squared test**. This test compares the observed frequencies against expected ones to calculate the test statistic.

The Chi- Squared (χ^2) statistic is compared against its critical value. If our test statistic value is larger than the critical value, we reject the null hypothesis (Figure 12.2).

The principle of this test can be utilised to conduct several different tests.

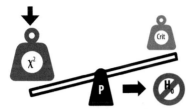

Figure 12.2 Reject H₀ when χ^2 statistic > critical value.

Chi-Squared Goodness of Fit Test

This test is known as the Chi-Squared **goodness of fit** test. We test the goodness of fit between the observed frequency against the expected frequency (Figure 12.3). When there is a significant discrepancy between the two, we reject H_0, i.e. we conclude that our observed frequencies have a **poor fit** to expected frequencies. The null hypothesis for χ^2 goodness of fit test is:

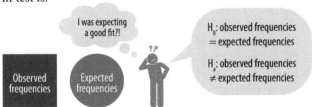

Figure 12.3 Goodness of fit test, comparing expected versus observed frequencies.

Let us assume we wish to investigate the customer satisfaction of a newly opened restaurant. We count the number of customers who are happy or sad on the day. We expected that 80% of customers would be happy and 20% sad. We had 25 customers on the day of whom only 15 were happy and 10 sad (Figure 12.4). If our hypothesis were correct, we would expect 20 happy customers and 5 sad customers. Was this just a chance variation? We calculate the χ^2 statistic (*the actual formula is given in the bonus section*). We find the critical value for the χ^2 statistic from the statistical table (**degrees of freedom (df) is k-1**, k is the number of levels of the categorical variables, in the above example it is 2-1=1). Our calculated χ^2 value is larger than the critical value, p = 0.012, the observed frequency of customer satisfaction did

Bullet Points

The Chi-Squared test is a **significance test.** It does not calculate an estimate.

The test is for **categorical** variables in **frequencies**.

It does *not* require distributional assumptions.

The Chi-Squared test compares **frequencies**, it **does not** test usual parameters like **mean**, median or Standard deviation.

Expected frequency: the frequency we **expect** to find if H_0 were **true**.

Bullet Points

Residual:

the **difference** between the observed frequency and the expected frequency.

Test statistic:

the sum total of the residual.

Null hypothesis in Chi-Squared test of independence:

the two categorical **variables** are **independent**.

not fit our expectation. This was not a chance variation, it was real, the restaurant performed poorly!

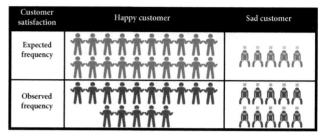

Figure 12.4 The Chi-Squared test, comparing observed versus expected frequency.

Chi-Squared Test of Independence/ Association

The ability of the Chi-Squared test to compare and contrast expected versus observed frequencies also allows us to test if two categorical variables are independent or related. If the variables are binary, they are best displayed in a **2 × 2 contingency** table (Figure 12.5), but larger tables can be used if one or both have >2 categories (**r x c** tables, **r** = number of *rows*, **c** = number of *columns*). Let us assume we are interested in investigating if passive smoking contributes to coronary death. It is usual practice to arrange the outcome (coronary death) in columns and the exposure in rows. The cohort is divided based on their exposure and outcome.

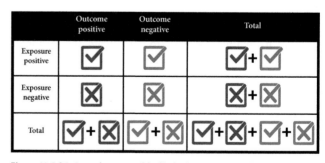

Figure 12.5 A 2x2 contingency table displaying exposure and outcome.

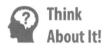

Think About It!

What does it mean when we say the variables are 'independent' of each other?

We surveyed 250 patients in total of whom 70 patients experienced coronary death (50 of them were passive smokers). One-hundred-and-eighty were alive, of whom 100 were passive smokers.. Let's put these data in Table 12.1.

	Outcome positive coronary death	Outcome negative No coronary death	Total
Exposure positive Passive smoking	50	100	150
Exposure negative No passive smoking	20	80	100
Total	70	180	250

Table 12.1 A 2 × 2 contingency table for passive smoking and coronary death.

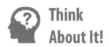

Think About It!

Do the sample sizes have to be equal for this test to be valid?

Our **null hypothesis** is:

The **row** variables and the **column** variables are **independent** (passive smoking status has no bearing on the risk of coronary death).

Degrees of freedom = (r-1) x (c-1), r = number of rows, c = number of columns . The *df* in a 2 × 2 contingency table is 1 (1 × 1).

How do we find the expected frequency? There is a formula for calculating expected frequency for the Chi-Squared test of independence:

What information do we gather regarding the strength of association from the Chi-Squared test?

$$\text{Expected cell frequency} = \frac{\text{Row total x Column total}}{n}$$

To calculate the expected frequency of each cell, we need to multiply the row and column totals for that cell and divide the product by the total number of cases in the table. Table 12.1 is reproduced below with the expected frequency and the method of calculation, p = 0.031, **we can reject H₀.**

Bullet Points

	Outcome positive coronary death	Outcome negative No coronary death	Total
Exposure positive Passive smoking	50 (42) (C1 × R1) ÷ n	100 (108) (C2 × R1) ÷ n	150 **(R1)**
Exposure negative No passive smoking	20 (28) (C1 × R2) ÷ n	80 (72) (C2 × R2) ÷ n	100 **(R2)**
Total	70 (C1)	180 (C2)	250 (n)

Table 12.2 Calculated (expected) frequencies.

Chi-Squared test for trend: when we test the association between a binominal variable and an ordinal categorical variable (e.g. degree of passive smoking).

Let Us Now See a Real-Life Example

Researchers were interested to learn if musculoskeletal symptoms were more prevalent in musicians compared

Is there a difference in outcome due to the different exposure categories, i.e. coronary death due to the severity of passive smoking?

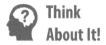

Think About It!

What does this test tell us about the cause–effect relationship?

What was the null hypothesis of this study?

Is the Chi-Squared test for independence a one- tailed or a two-tailed test?

to non-musicians given their need to frequently repeat physically strenuous movements [3]. They undertook a cross-sectional study. The table below shows a difference in apparent prevalence rate between the musicians and non-musicians. Is this for real? To test this the authors conducted the χ^2 test. The test would assume that there was no relationship between being a musician and having musculoskeletal symptoms. Comparing the test statistic against the degree of freedom they concluded that there was **< 0.1% chance** that the observed difference in musculoskeletal symptoms in the elbow, wrist and hand region over the last 12 months between the musicians and non-musicians (48.2% versus 22%) could have been due to chance alone. The **null hypothesis** was **disproved** (musician and musculoskeletal complaints are not independent). The authors concluded that musculoskeletal complaints were significantly more common among musicians compared to non-musicians. There was no significant difference in lower back complaints between the two groups (Table 12.3).

Body region	Complaints	Musical students n=83	Medical students n=494	Difference (p-value)
Elbow, wrist, hand	in the last 12 months	40 (48.2%)	109 (22%)	p <0.001
Lower back	in the last 12 months	33 (39.8%)	191 (39%)	p = 0.860

Table. 12.3 Data from Kok et al. [3].

Do We Get Any Information about the Effect Size?

We get no information about the effect size from the Chi-Squared test. This is simply a test of the null hypothesis and only informs us whether or not there is a relationship between the column variable and the row variable.

Bullet Points

McNemar's test: when samples are matched (not independent).

So far, we have learnt how to perform a significance test involving different types of variables. Let us learn in the next chapter how to test for association between numerical variables.

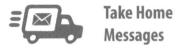

Take Home Messages

• The Chi-Squared test is performed when we have frequencies in categories.

• The expected frequency refers to the frequency we expect to see if the null hypothesis were correct.

• The test compares the observed frequency against the expected frequency to calculate the χ^2 statistic.

• The χ^2 statistic is compared along with the degrees of freedom against the χ^2 distribution to find the critical value of the statistic.

• If the calculated χ^2 statistic is larger than the critical value, we reject the null hypothesis.

• There are several χ^2 tests: test for goodness of fit, test of association and test for trend.

• The null hypothesis of the χ^2 goodness of fit test is that there is no difference between the observed frequency and the expected frequency.

• We utilise a contingency table to perform the χ^2 test of independence.

• The null hypothesis of the χ^2 test of independence is that the column variables and the row variables are independent.

• The χ^2 test of independence compares the cell counts of the observed frequency against the expected frequency.

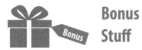

Bonus Stuff

What Is the Formula for the Chi-Squared Test?

$$\chi^2 = \Sigma \frac{(O - E)^2}{E}$$

O = observed frequency
E = expected frequency
Σ = sum of all cells

Do We Need to Make any Assumptions for the Chi-Squared Test to Be Valid?

Yes, the observations are independent, i.e. each subject contributed data to only one cell and there are no repeated observations. It is assumed that observations are collected on a random basis. Data must be in frequencies and not in percentage or proportions. It is a test of numbers. As the frequencies become smaller, the difference between the expected and the observed frequencies become less so and the test becomes less powerful. For the test to be valid at least 80% of *expected* frequencies must be >5 and all expected frequencies >1 [4]. Note *expected*, not observed.

Why Do I See Yates' Correction and Fisher's Exact Test in Some Papers?

Confusingly for us, the χ^2 distribution is a square of the Standard normal distribution and hence a continuous distribution [5]. Extrapolation of results of a discrete probability to a continuous distribution may introduce some error. Many recommend the use of **Yates' continuity correction** in a 2 × 2 table, even when sample size requirements are met to help reduce this error. Altman recommends it for *all* Chi-Squared tests on *2x2 tables* [5]. The argument for using the Yates' correction is to reduce the risk of type I error.

However, the test has been criticised for being too conservative and increasing the risk for type II error. Many statisticians feel that it is unnecessary [6]. Kirkwood and Sterne commented that it makes *little* difference unless *the total sample size is <40* [7]. On the other hand, if sample size assumptions are not met, the Chi-Squared test may not be valid. Cochran recommends *Fisher's exact test* instead when the *total sample is <20, or the overall total is 20-40 and the smallest of the four expected numbers <5* [7]. There is no sample size restriction for Fisher's exact test. The detailed calculation of the exact test is beyond the scope of our discussion.

Questions & Answers

Q: What does it mean when we say the variables are 'independent' of each other?

A: It means that one variable predicts nothing about the other variable, i.e. knowing a person is a passive smoker gives us no clue about the likely coronary death of that person compared to a non-passive smoker. This is akin to H_0: there is no difference in coronary death between passive smokers and non-passive smokers (i.e. the frequency of coronary death does not vary between the two groups). The test is also known as a test of association, i.e. there is no association between the two variables.

Q: Do the sample sizes have to be equal for this test to be valid?

A: There is no need for the sample sizes to be equal (there was no need for an equal number of participants with positive and negative exposure to passive smoking).

Q: What information do we gather regarding the strength of association from the Chi-Squared test?

A: The Chi-Squared test is simply a hypothesis test and gives no idea about the strength of association.

Q: What does this test tell us about the cause–effect relationship?

A: The test simply comments on the statistical significance of the relationship between two variables, not whether there is a cause–effect relationship.

Q: What was the null hypothesis in this study?

A: The researchers were interested to know if musculoskeletal symptoms were more prevalent in musicians compared to non-musicians. The null hypothesis was that being a musician had no bearing on musculoskeletal symptoms, the two variables were completely independent of each other.

Q: Is the Chi-Squared test for independence a one-tailed or a two-tailed test?

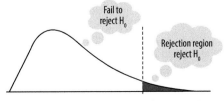

Figure 12.6: H_0 is only rejected when χ^2 statistic is large and positive.

A: All χ^2 tests are one-tailed. We are only interested to find out if the χ^2 statistic is way-off to the right to indicate a poor fit, we are not interested to find out if the statistic indicates too good a fit. For the χ^2 statistic to be significant to reject H_0, it has to be positive (Figure 12.6).

CHAPTER 13

If the Line Fits
Correlation and Linear Regression

In other words, it must be concluded that there is a real association between carcinoma of the lung and smoking.

Doll and Hill

Did You Know?

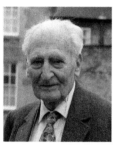

© CJ DUB CC ASA2 [1].

Figure 13.1 Sir William Richard Doll CH, OBE, FRS (1912–2005), was a British physician and a pioneering epidemiologist. Working along with Sir Bradford Hill, he found the link between smoking and lung cancer. He subsequently initiated the prospective **British Doctors' study** that ran for half a century and confirmed his initial findings as well as many other harmful effects of smoking [2].

🎯 Learning Outcomes

We shall discuss the following material in this chapter:
• How do we test for linear correlation between continuous variables
• What is a correlation coefficient
• Why correlation is not necessarily causation
• What is the difference between correlation and linear regression
• What is the advantage of multiple linear regression

Linear Correlation

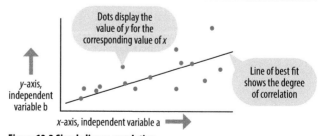

Figure 13.2 Simple linear correlation.

In the previous chapter, we learnt how to test for the relationship between categorical variables. When both dependent and independent variables are continuous and we want to investigate if there is a linear relationship between them, we investigate **correlation**. The first step to testing this relationship is to collect data and plot them in a scatterplot. Data are displayed as a collection of points in a scatterplot.

A scatterplot allows a visual inspection of the relation between the variables. Once data are plotted, a line can be drawn through the points to assess the extent of the linear correlation. Let us see an example [3]. The Japanese are famous for their long lifespan. Researchers observed that old Japanese men seem to have large ears. They wondered if lifespan had any relation to ear length. Data were collected for participants aged 20-94. The authors plotted age in the *x*-axis and ear length in the *y*-axis. Figure 13.2 shows an example of a simple linear correlation graph. Data fit reasonably well in a straight line with an upward slope in the above graph. This is a sign of a **positive linear correlation**. Figure 13.3 illustrates different degrees of correlation.

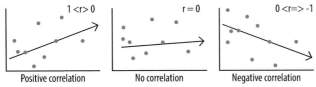

Figure 13.3 Different degrees of linear correlation.

How Strong Is the Correlation?

The researchers established that there was a positive linear correlation between ear length and age, but how strong was this relation? To find the answer, we need to quantify the strength of the relationship through a statistical measure. This is known as *r* or **Pearson's correlation coefficient**. Pearson's coefficient is a measure of how much the *two variables move together* or *how closely* the points lie to the straight line, *not* the **gradient** of the line. An *r*-value of **0** means **no** correlation, a value of **1** indicates a **perfect positive** correlation and a value of −1 indicates a **perfect negative** correlation. An *r*-value of >0.8 indicates a strong positive correlation. The correlation coefficient of ear length with age was 0.30 (95% CI 0.21 to 0.39) [3]. This suggests that both variables moved in the **same direction** (ear length increased with increasing age) The researchers were correct!

Bullet Points

Correlation:
to test the strength of *linear* relation between **numerical** exposure and outcome variables. **Discrete or ordinal data** can also be assessed.

Sample correlation coefficient: *r*

Population correlation coefficient: ρ

Correlation in numbers:

1: perfect *positive* correlation (both variables move in the *same* direction)

0: no correlation

-1: perfect *negative* correlation (variables move in the *opposite* direction)

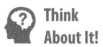

Think About It!

What is the unit of correlation?

How would you know if the relationship between the variables was non-linear?

What would be the null hypothesis of a significance test for correlation coefficient?

What is the likely relation of ear length to age in a person aged <20 or >94 years?

Was This Genuine or Just a Fluke?

We don't know if this relationship was real or just a chance finding. To confirm this, we need to calculate the p-value. Note that the authors did not cite a p-value since they provided us with 95% CI. The range of the CI did not include 0, therefore, the relationship was statistically significant, not a fluke.

Does Old Age Cause Big Ears?

Our findings confirmed that ear length increased with increasing age, but not that increasing age caused longer ears! Just because we found a correlation between the two variables does not mean one caused the other. **Correlation is not causation**, even if the relationship is valid. There is evidence of a valid positive correlation between ice cream sales and homicide rate but enjoying ice cream does not turn one into a homicidal maniac [4]. Both happen to increase in summer.

Be Careful of Spurious Correlation

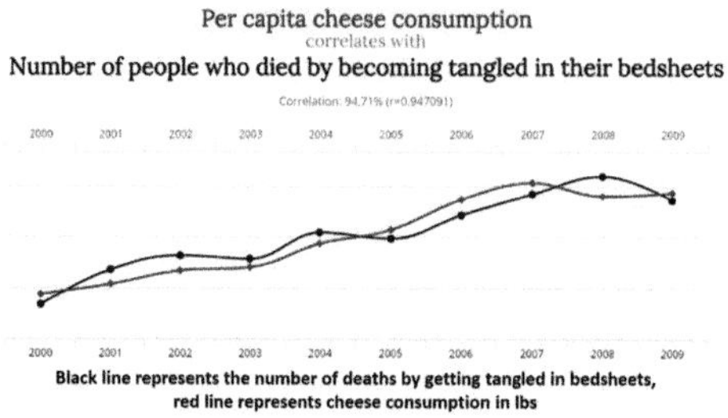

Per capita cheese consumption
correlates with
Number of people who died by becoming tangled in their bedsheets

Correlation: 94.71% (r=0.947091)

Black line represents the number of deaths by getting tangled in bedsheets, red line represents cheese consumption in lbs

Figure 13.4 Spurious correlation between cheese consumption and death.
© Spurious correlations, reproduced under the CC licence.

It is possible to find a statistical correlation that does not make sense in real life by looking for opportunistic chance associations. The website **Spurious correlations** is an excellent online source that uses real-life data to demonstrate the futility of making apparently sound statistical correlations that do not make practical sense. Here is an example (Figure 13.4) [5]. The graph suggests that the US per capita cheese consumption correlated with the number of people who died by getting entangled in bedsheets!

Linear Regression: If the Line Fits!

Linear correlation coefficient informed us that both age and ear length moved in the same direction but did not allow us to **predict** by how much. We need to conduct a **linear regression** equation to answer this question. The researchers commented [3]:

> The linear regression equation between age and ear length was: ear length = 61.8+(0.13 x age) (95% CI for the regression coefficient 0.09 to 0.17).

They conducted a **linear regression** analysis and were able to quantify the linear relation. Ear length was the dependent variable, age was the independent variable. This is a regression of year (in age) to ear length (in mm). The equation is useful to predict ear length. The slope of the gradient is 0.13. It is the amount (in mm) of change in ear length for each year of age. 61.8 is the intercept, it is the value of ear length when age is set at 0. Here a **single variable** has been used to predict the outcome of the dependent variable. This kind of analysis is also known as a **Simple linear regression (SLR)**. If we wish to **include multiple independent variables** in our model, we need to perform a **multiple linear regression**.

The Line of Best Fit: The Least Square Method

The linear regression line is drawn employing a technique known as the least square method. Essentially all possible straight lines are considered, and the difference in height (**residual**) from the lines to the data points in the scatterplots are calculated. The line is chosen that shows the best fit of all (Figure 13.5). The best fit of line should have the minimum (least) sum of squared residuals. The **formula for the SLR is:** $y = \alpha + \beta x$ where α is the intercept or constant and is the value of y when x is 0 and β is the slope (increase in y for each unit increase in x). R^2 is an estimate of **goodness of fit** of the model and is the square of Pearson's correlation coefficient, expressed in percentage. In the example above relating to age and ear length, the R^2 value was $(0.30)^2 = 0.09 \times 100\% = 9\%$. The R^2 value indicates that only 9% of the variation in ear length could be explained by its variation due to age.

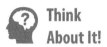

Think About It!

Can you predict from this model how age will change with change in ear length?

What is the difference between correlation and linear regression?

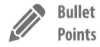

Bullet Points

Linear regression: to predict the relationship between a numerical outcome and exposure.

Formula for simple linear regression: $y = \alpha + \beta x$

Simple: single independent variable.

Multiple: multiple independent variables.

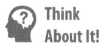

**Think
About It!**

If the values of *r* are low, does it necessarily mean that there is no relation between the variables?

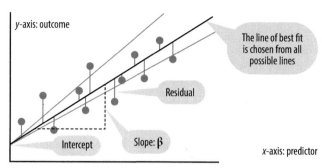

Figure 13.5 Drawing the line of best fit by minimising the vertical distances above and below the line.

Is there any difference between conducting multiple simple linear regression and multiple linear regression?

Correlation or Linear Regression: When Do I Use Which?

Correlation and linear regression both are measures of a linear relationship between two variables but are different. Correlation coefficient indicates *whether there is a linear relationship* and if so in which direction. If we wish to quantify this and *predict* to what extent a unit change in the independent variable affects the dependent variable, we need to perform a *Linear regression*.

Let us see an example. Researchers were interested to investigate the relationship between several radiological parameters after wrist fracture. They collected their data, displayed them in a scatterplot, visually established a linear relationship, performed a correlation coefficient to assess the strength of this relationship and finally performed linear regression to predict the behaviour of the dependent variable [6]:

> Linear regression analysis was performed to investigate the relationship between measures of carpal alignment and dorsal tilt. This method was chosen after scatterplots demonstrated a linear relationship between the variables. We created individual linear regression models for each measurement at each of the three times when radiographs were performed (initial, after reduction and final).

So far, we have learnt how to assess and interpret simple (single) linear regression. Let us now see how we can assess and control for the influence of multiple variables at the same time.

**Bullet
Points**

Linear regression and correlation **both** have their uses. Linear **correlation** informs us how one variable *changes* the other but not *how closely they are related*. We need to calculate **regression** to quantify this relation.

Multiple Linear Regression

Multiple linear regression (MLR) can simultaneously assess the contribution of several variables. It can, therefore, adjust for the differences in the effect of these variables and thus control for confounding. In MLR, the independent variables can be a mix of numerical and categorical ones, the dependent variable needs to be continuous. Let us see an example; researchers were interested to investigate how morphological abnormality of the hip joint affected sleep quality [7]. They measured sleep quality with a 21-point Pittsburgh Sleep Quality Index (PSQI) Scale (higher PSQI scores indicate worse sleep quality). Patients completed questionnaires that included the Hip disability and Osteoarthritis Outcome Score (HOOS), Short Form Health Survey (SF-12). Below is an extract from the results (Table 13.1). The model suggests that after adjusting for several confounders sleep quality was significantly affected by HOOS pain, SF-12 role emotional and SF-12 mental health subscales.

Model outcome and predictors	Mean estimate	95% CI
PSQI total		
Intercept	20.2082	17.0903 to 23.4622
HOOS pain	−0.0794	−0.01150 to −0.0430
SF-12 role emotional	−0.0817	−0.1405 to −0.0320
SF-12 mental health	−0.0653	−0.1263 to −0.0199

Table 13.1 Sleep quality and nocturnal pain, from Reddy et al. [7].
© BMC Musculoskeletal Disorders, reproduced under the CC licence.

The range of the CI confirms that all the variables listed are significantly predictive of the outcome. A patient with a low score in SF-12 role emotional scale would have poor sleep irrespective of the mental health or pain level. The intercept indicates the PSQI score when all the independent variables are set to zero. The regression coefficient suggests that for each unit increase in HOOS pain scale (higher score indicates less hip pain) there was a 0.0794-unit reduction in PSQI scale (sleep quality improved with improvement in pain) independent of other factors. The adjusted R^2 value was 0.404, confirming that 40% of the variation in sleep quality could be explained by the model.

In the next chapter, we shall learn how to perform a logistic regression analysis to predict the outcome of binary variables.

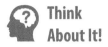

Think About It!

What part of the regression line does the regression coefficient represent?

What is the likely probable range of R^2 value?

Bullet Points

Multiple Linear Regression (MLR):
single numerical dependent variable, *multiple* independent variables.

Regression coefficient in MLR:
the mean change in the dependent variable for each unit change in the independent variable when *all other* independent variables are *constant.*

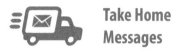

Take Home Messages

• When we wish to investigate for a linear relationship between continuous variables, we plot the variables in a scatterplot and find the line of best fit.

• Pearson's correlation coefficient r helps us to quantify the strength of the linear relationship.

• The possible values of Pearson's correlation coefficient range from −1 to +1.

• An r-score of +1 means a perfect positive correlation, 0 means no correlation and -1 means perfect negative correlation.

• If an r-score is 0, it does not mean there is no relationship, simply that there is no linear relationship.

• Just because there is a correlation does not mean one variable causes the other variable to change: correlation does not mean causation.

• Linear regression is necessary to quantify the linear relationship and develop a predictive model.

• The R^2 value is an estimate of the goodness of fit of the regression model and is the square of Pearson's correlation coefficient, expressed in a percentage.

• Multiple linear regression can assess for the influence of multiple independent variables at the same time and thus control for the effect of confounding factors.

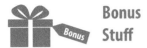

Bonus Stuff

More about Correlation Coefficients

Pearson's correlation coefficient requires a distributional assumption. At least one of the numerical variables must follow a normal distribution. If a numerical variable does not follow the normal distribution, we need to calculate **Spearman's rank correlation coefficient** instead. Spearman's test can also be performed if one of the variables is an ordinal one or the relationship is non-linear. Alternatively, **Kendall's correlation coefficient** test can also be performed.

What Is the Residual?

The residual is the vertical difference in height between the observed and the predicted value of the dependent variable. It is the error in the prediction of the model (Figure 13.5).

What Are the Assumptions Required for a Valid Linear Regression Analysis?

Several assumptions need to be satisfied for linear regression to be valid:

• The relationship between the independent and the dependent variables is linear.

• The residuals are independent and normally distributed (note *residuals*, not data).

• The variance of y is the same at each value of x or the relationship between the two variables stays the same at all points.

• Multiple independent variables should not be related. If they are correlated, appropriate adjustments need to be made in the model in the form of interaction terms.

How Do I Decide Which Variables to Include in a Multiple Regression Model?

A widely accepted method is to perform univariable analysis first and include only the significant variables in the MLR model. MLR should not be attempted for small datasets but textbooks do not indicate any minimum sample size.

Questions & Answers

Q: What is the unit of correlation?

A: Correlation has no units. It is a measure of linear association between two variables between a score of -1 to +1.

Q: How would you know if the relationship between variables were non-linear?

A: Pearson's correlation coefficient only investigates a linear relationship and will not be able to identify a non-linear relationship. When the variables are plotted, visual inspection would indicate a non-linear relationship.

Q: What would be the null hypothesis of a significance test for the correlation coefficient?

A: The correlation coefficient only investigates a linear relationship. Therefore, the H_0 is: there is no linear relationship between the two variables. The H_a is: there is a linear relationship between the two variables.

Q: Looking back at the correlation of the age and ear length of Japanese men, what is the likely relation of ear length to age in a person aged <20 or >94 years?

A: It is not possible to extrapolate results beyond the available data in correlation. Since no one in the observed study was aged <20 or >94 years, it is not possible to predict the relationship between ear length and age in someone aged <20 or >94 years. Similarly, when we model linear regression the value of the dependent variable (y-axis) cannot be extrapolated beyond the available values of the independent variable (x-axis) used in the model.

Q: Can you predict from this model how age will change with change in ear length?

A: No, it is not possible to predict a change in age from a change in ear length. The estimate was calculated specifically for change in ear length with age, the calculation cannot be reversed.

Q: What is the difference between correlation and linear regression?

A: Correlation is an indication of the strength of the linear relationship between two variables: strongly positive (score near to 1), weakly positive (score near to 0), no relation (score of 0), weakly negative (score near to 0), strongly negative (score near to −1), etc. Linear regression is also a measure of linear correlation. It is complementary to correlation. Linear regression does not look at the strength of relation; instead, it predicts the value of the dependent variable for a given value of the independent variable.

Q: If the value of r is low, does it necessarily mean that there is no relation between the variables?

A: The role of correlation coefficient r is only to assess if there is a linear relation. Therefore, even if the value of r is low it does not mean there is no relation, simply that there is no evidence of a linear relationship, it may well be that there is a non-linear relationship.

Q: Is there any difference between conducting multiple single linear regression and multiple linear regression?

A: Yes, there is a difference. Simple linear regression is not able to control for the effect of confounders. When multiple simple linear regression analyses are performed, they would confirm the relation of multiple independent variables concerning the dependent variable in isolation, but will not be able to inform us how they perform together. This information would only be available after a multiple linear regression analysis.

Q: What part of the regression line does the regression coefficient represent?

A: The regression coefficient represents the gradient of the regression line.

Q: What is the likely probable range of the R^2 value?

A: The probable range of the R^2 value can only lie between 0-1. Zero indicates that the model is not at all predictive and 1 indicates a perfect prediction.

CHAPTER 14

Hindsight is 20/20
Logistic Regression

> We shall not insist on the hypothesis of geometric progression, given that it can hold only in very special circumstances.
>
> **P. Verhulst**

Did You Know?

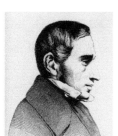

© Public domain [1].

Figure 14.1 Pierre F. Verhulst (1804–1849), was a Belgian mathematician. He developed the Logistic function while trying to prove that population growth did not follow geometric progression as suggested by Malthus. He died at a young age due to poor health a year after being elected the President of the Belgian Academy of Sciences [2].

Learning Outcomes

We shall discuss the following material in this chapter:
- Logistic regression and how it works
- Simple and multiple logistic regression: the difference
- The Logit function and the sigmoid curve
- Interpreting the results of the logistic regression
- What does the Wald statistic inform us of
- Why do we need the Hosmer and Lemeshow test
- The Nagelkerke R^2 and how to interpret it
- Why we should not forget the minimum event rule

Introduction to Logistic Regression

In the previous chapter, we learnt how to create a linear regression model using single or multiple independent variables to predict the outcome of a continuous variable. When our outcome of interest is **binary**, we perform the **Logistic regression** analysis. The independent or explanatory variables can be numerical or categorical. The model can be simple – when we utilise a single independent variable, e.g. predicting lung cancer from smoking habit, or multiple – when we utilise several independent variables, e.g. predicting lung cancer from smoking history, family history, occupation, exposure to passive smoking etc. Since the outcome is binary it can't be modelled on a linear scale; the **logistic model** uses a **sigmoid curve** or a **big** S-shaped line

(Figure 14.2). When we plot the independent variable in a chart, the model predicts the probability of the independent variable predicting the binary outcome. The outcome is either **1** (**true**, present) or **0** (**false**, absent).

Bullet Points

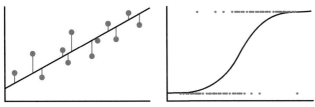

Figure 14.2 Comparing linear versus logistic regression.

The *odds* of outcome are modelled on a *logarithmic* scale.

Log odds of the outcome is the **Logit** function.

Let us see an example (Figure 14.3). Here smoking is the exposure variable and lung cancer the outcome. If the **probability of lung cancer is >50%** on the sigmoid curve, the **outcome** is classified as **1** (lung cancer present); if the likelihood is <**50%** it is **0** (no lung cancer). To avoid the limitation of having to model a binary outcome the outcome is transformed and calculated on a log scale. The transformation of the outcome or the log (odds) is the *logit* function and the model is known as *Logistic* regression. Logit function can calculate any value for the *y*-axis despite it being a binary variable. *We have not discussed odds yet; we shall learn more about them in the next chapter.*

Probability in **Logistic regression**: 0 *or* 1.

Types of logistic regression:

Single **outcome**: uni**variate**

Multiple **outcomes**: multi**variate**

Single independent *variable*: uni*variable*

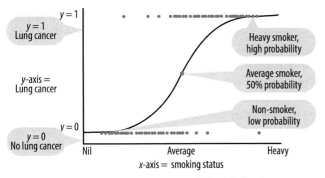

Figure 14.3 A graphical illustration explaining the logistic function.

Multiple independent *variables*: multi*variable*

Note the **difference** between multi*variate* and multi*variable*.

How Do You Fit the Line in Logistic Regression?

We do not use the least squares method and do not calculate residuals in logistic regression. In the least squares method, we tried to minimise the distance between the data points and the best line of fit. In logistic regression, we use the

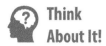

Think About It!

What type of model has been discussed in the example?

What is the difference between the Chi-Squared test and Logistic regression?

What should you suspect if you notice a large difference in crude OR and adjusted OR in your model?

What would be the advantage of conducting Logistic regression analyses in case-control studies?

maximum likelihood method, whereby we try to calculate the different types of a sigmoid curve from the various data points. The curve that has the maximum likelihood of fitting the data is chosen, i.e. the line is optimised to fit the data best. **Logistic regression** finds the **equation** that **best predicts** the value of *y* **from** *x* via the **sigmoid curve**.

Let Us See an Example

Hip fracture is a major public health hazard with a high mortality rate. Researchers were interested to investigate if the time to surgery affected 30-day mortality. The outcome was a binary one: alive or dead 30 days after hip fracture. The authors commented [3]:

> Age, gender, pre-fracture mobility, MMTS and ASA grade were statistically significant predictors of 30-day mortality on [...] binary logistic regression.

We note that more than one independent variable was used. This is known as **multivariable logistic regression** and is akin to multiple linear regression. Initially, the authors performed univariable analysis and variables found to be significant were analysed together in the multivariable model. Several factors that were predictive of 30-day mortality were found to be no longer significant in the multivariable analysis (Table 14.1). The probability is expressed in Odds ratios (OR). OR can vary from 0 to infinity. OR>1 means the event is more likely and OR<1 means the event is less likely. From the table we conclude that all things being equal, 30-day mortality will *increase* **2.5 times** (adjusted OR 2.5) for **each grade** *increase* in **ASA** status. Thirty-day mortality will *increase* by **3.9% for each year** (OR 1.039). Being **female** will *reduce* mortality by (1-0.725= 0.275) or **27.5%**. For **each grade** *increase* in **mobility** score, mortality will be **reduced** by (1-0.925= 0.075) or **7.5%**.

	Wald	p-value	Adjusted OR
Age	21.479	<0.001	1.039
Female gender	6.072	0.014	0.725
ASA grade	93.561	<0.001	2.517
Mobility score	6.08	0.014	0.925

Table 14.1 Extract from the multivariable logistic regression model [3].

What about the Wald Statistic?

In the table above, we noted the Wald statistic in the second column. It is a test to see if individual independent variables in the model are useful. This is done by assessing the statistical significance of their regression coefficient. If the value is significant, the variable adds useful value to the model and should be included. A value that is not significant is not useful to the model. All the variables above were significant.

What Is the Significance of the Hosmer and Lemeshow Test and the Nagelkerke R^2 Value?

The authors further commented [3]:

> The Hosmer–Lemeshow test denoted a good model fit (chi-squared test, chi = 5.468, p = 0.707). The variables included in the model predicted 13.1% of the variance in 30-day mortality (Nagelkerke r-square = 0.131)[...] The validity of the model was upheld with 402 events (deaths within 30 days of admission).

The Hosmer and Lemeshow test is a test of the *lack of fit* of the model [4]. The test calculates the difference between the number of observed and expected events. If the difference is high, the agreement is poor, and the p-value is significant. If the difference is low, the p-value is high and not significant. In the above example, we saw that the p-value was 0.707 suggesting that there was **no evidence** of a **lack of goodness** of fit.

There are several ways to assess the predictive power of the model, these are known as **pseudo R^2**. The pseudo R^2 value is a measure of how well we can predict the dependent variable from the model variables. **Nagelkerke R^2** is one of them. The R^2 value above suggests that the model would account for 13% of the variability in 30-day mortality.

Why Do We Need a Minimum Event Rule?

The authors further commented that the model was valid because it had 402 events. What does it mean? The reliability

Bullet Points

How could we know how good the model is?

There is *no* single indicator, **goodness of fit and predictive power** should both be stated when the model is discussed [5].

Hosmer and Lemeshow test:

H_0: the model has *lack of goodness of fit*

High p-value is *good*, model has good fit.

Adjusted Odds Ratios: Odds Ratios that adjust for other predictor variables in a multivariable model. *Adjusted OR is further explained in the Bonus Stuff section.*

Bullet Points

When the independent variable has >2 categories OR is calculated for the baseline category and each different category.

The non-baseline categories are known as **indicator** or **dummy** variables.

of a model diminishes with smaller sample sizes. As a rule of thumb, it is suggested that there should be at least ten events for every predictor variable [6]. There were 402 deaths and seven predictors in the model, the number of events was adequate.

Tell Us about the Indicator Variable

If the independent variable is categorical and has >2 categories we have to indicate to the software that the variable is *categorical* and create a baseline category as well as **indicator** or **dummy** variables for other categories (k-1 indicator variables created for k categories). The model will calculate the OR for each category compared to the baseline. While assessing the risk of lung cancer from exposure to smoking, we might denote nil smoking as the baseline category and create indicator variables for average (smoking^1) and heavy smoking (smoking^2). The model will calculate the OR of lung cancer for average and heavy smoking compared to the nil smoking category.

Is Logistic Regression Assumption-Free?

Did You Know?

Logistic regression is widely used for machine learning algorithms and artificial intelligence.

Logistic regression requires that the observations are independent and there is a linear relationship between the logit function of the dependent variable and the independent continuous variable. The independent variables should be independent of each other and not correlated, this is known as *multicollinearity*. When multicollinearity is present it can affect the precision of the model. A detailed discussion is beyond our scope, but a reading list is included for those interested in *Appendix 4.*

We briefly discussed odds of an outcome and learnt how and why logistic regression model calculates Odds ratios for binary outcomes. Let's learn more about them in the next chapter.

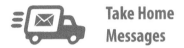

Take Home Messages

- Logistic regression is used to investigate a binary outcome.

- The model is known as *logistic* because it is fitted on a *logarithmic* scale, the odds of an outcome are modelled on a logarithmic scale.

- Logit function is the log odds of the outcome.

- The model can be univariate (to investigate a single outcome) or multivariate (multiple outcomes), univariable (single independent variable) or multivariable (multiple independent variables).

- Instead of a straight line, logistic regression uses a sigmoid curve.

- The sigmoid curve is fitted using the maximum likelihood method.

- The output of logistic regression is displayed as Odds ratios.

- Multiple logistic regression can control for the effects of confounders.

- Multiple logistic regression gives an adjusted odds ratio.

- The Wald statistic is calculated to test whether individual predictive variables are significant.

- The Hosmer and Lemeshow test is a test of lack of goodness of fit of the regression model.

- The Nagelkerke R^2 value is a measure of how well we can predict the dependent variable from the model.

- The minimum event rule of thumb is that there should be at least ten events for every predictor variable included in the model.

- When the *independent* variable has more than two categories a baseline category is indicated and several indicator or dummy variables are created to identify the different categories in relation to a baseline reference category. Probability of events and OR are calculated for each indicator variable compared to the reference category.

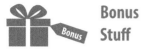

Bonus Stuff

More about the Logit Function

The logit function is the log of the ratio of the probabilities.
p = the probability of an event taking place,
1-p = the probability of the event not taking place.

$$\text{Logit function} = \text{logit}(p) = \text{Log} \frac{p}{1-p}$$

What Is the Difference between the Unadjusted and the Adjusted Odds Ratios?

When we perform univariable logistic regression the resultant Odds ratios (OR) gives us an estimate based on a single independent variable. The model cannot adjust for the effects of other confounders, they were never there in the model. However, when we perform a multivariable logistic regression the model takes into account the dynamics between several independent predictors and the estimated OR adjusts for the simultaneous effects of multiple independent variables. This is known as the adjusted OR.

The difference between the adjusted and the unadjusted OR gives us an idea about the extent of confounding. A multivariable model is more akin to a real-life scenario. In life, it is rare for a single exposure variable to have a clear relationship with the outcome in a way that its effect is not modified by other predictor variables. Even though smoking is an obvious risk factor for lung cancer, other factors like passive smoking, occupational exposure, family history etc. also modify its effect but this may not always be the case.

Here is an example, since both systemic steroid use and habitual alcohol intake are major risk factors for idiopathic osteonecrosis of the femoral head (ONFH), researchers wished to investigate their effect on the risk of ONFH. The results suggested that compared to non-drinkers, subjects with ≥ 3032 drink-years had a crude OR of 2.53 for ONFH (adjusted OR 3.93). This would suggest that compared to non-drinkers, patients with alcohol intake ≥ 3032 drink-years were 2.5 times more likely to develop ONFH. However, the risk was nearly four-times as likely when adjusted for the effect of potential confounders [7].

Therefore, non-drinkers had other confounding risk factors that masked the true risk of ONFH from drinking. When these factors were taken into account, all things being equal, the actual risk of ONFH from drinking was higher than initially suspected.

Questions & Answers

Q: What type of model has been discussed in the study investigating the relationship of time to surgery to 30-day mortality following hip fracture?

A: It is a univariate (30-day mortality) multivariable (multiple independent variables) logistic model.

Q: What is the difference between the Chi-Squared test and logistic regression?

A: Both the Chi-Squared test and the logistic regression test are used to test categorical variables. However, the Chi-Squared test is a test of association only. The test does not have any predictive power. Logistic regression is also used in categorical variables, but it is a modelling technique and can be used to predict the outcome of a dependent variable from independent variables. If the purpose is just to investigate a relationship between two binary variables, the Chi-Squared test is adequate; if the aim is to predict the dependent variable, then Logistic regression is required.

Q: What should you suspect if you notice a large difference in crude OR and adjusted OR in your model?

A: Let us remember that the purpose of adjusted OR is to minimise the effect of confounding. Therefore, a large difference between the crude OR and the adjusted OR would suggest the likely presence of confounding factors in the model.

Q: What would be the advantage of conducting Logistic regression analyses in case-control studies?

A: In a case-control study, the outcome is already predetermined, and controls are recruited to match the cases. Since cases and controls are purposefully recruited and not random, the sample is not representative of the actual population at risk. Therefore, calculation of risk is not valid; OR is the only valid marker of the probability of event rate, and this is calculated by Logistic regression. Due to the sampling technique, even if the samples are matched, there is scope for confounding. Logistic regression analysis is an excellent technique to minimise the effect of confounding, although it is better to control it with a careful study design.

CHAPTER 15

Don't Risk the Odds
Risk versus Odds as the Outcome Measure

Did You Know?

A dispute between gamblers in a dice game in 1654 led to Blaise Pascal and Pierre de Fermat developing the probability theory.

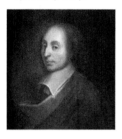

© CCA 3.0 [1].

Figure 15.1a Blaise Pascal (1623–1662), was a French mathematician and one of the first to develop a mechanical calculator [2].

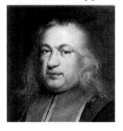

© Public domain [3].

Figure 15.1b Pierre de Fermat (1607–1665), is best known for *Fermat's last theorem* [4].

Thus, joining the rigor of demonstrations in mathematics with the uncertainty of chance, and conciliating these apparently contradictory matters, it can, taking its name from both of them, with justice arrogate the stupefying name: The Mathematics of Chance.   **Blaise Pascal**

 Learning Outcomes

We shall discuss the following material in this chapter:
• The difference between risk and odds
• How to calculate them
• What is relative risk
• Odds versus risk ratios
• The difference between relative and absolute risk
• The number needed to treat and harm
• When is it appropriate to use odds as the outcome measure

'How you can lower your diabetes risk by 22% just by looking out the window' [5], claimed a news headline. *'Blood clot risk doubles for some new contraceptive pills,'* said another [6]. News about odds and risks are regularly sensationalised in the national media. What lends them to such hype?

Risk versus Odds

Previously we learnt how to construct a 2x2 contingency table for binary variables and to investigate whether the two variables are significantly related. When we examine binary variables, we can also calculate the relative likelihood of events taking place. We express this probability by the terms **risk** and **odds**.

Odds and risks *both* calculate the **probability** of an *event*. However, there are some crucial differences between them. We can visualise from Figure 15.2 that **risk** is the proportion of patients in the whole population who experience the event. We calculate risk by dividing the *number of events* by the *entire* population at risk. **Odds** indicate the probability of an event taking place versus it not taking place. We calculate odds of an event by dividing the *number of events* by the *number of non-events* in the population at risk.

Bullet Points

Risk in medical statistics is the **probability** of an event in a population.

Risk: does not *always* imply a negative outcome.

$$\textbf{Risk}: \quad \frac{\text{Number of events}}{\text{Population at risk}}$$

$$\textbf{Odds}: \quad \frac{\text{Number of events}}{\text{Number of non-events}}$$

Range of probability:

0–1: 0 is none, 1 is 100;

this is expressed in percentages = (probability x 100) 0.3 probability = 0.3 x 100 = 30% probability.

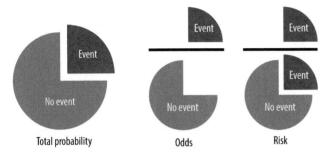

Figure 15.2 Calculation of risk versus odds, difference is in the *denominator*!

Let us see an example. Researchers wished to investigate if cholesterol-lowering with simvastatin in patients with pre-existing coronary heart disease (CHD) affected coronary (CVD) death [7]. Four thousand four hundred and forty-four patients were randomised to a double-blind trial with simvastatin or placebo. There were 189 coronary deaths in the placebo group and 111 in the simvastatin group. Let us look at these numbers through a 2 × 2 contingency table (Table 15.1) (*data from the Scandinavian Simvastatin Survival Study*)[7].

CVD death	No death	Population at risk
Statin: 111	2064 (46 non CVD death)	2221
Placebo: 189	1985 (49 non CVD death)	2223

Table 15.1 Coronary (CVD) death in statin versus placebo.

$$\frac{\textbf{Risk} \text{ of CVD death}}{\text{in the } \textbf{statin} \text{ group}} = \frac{\text{Event in exposed}}{\text{Total at risk}} = \frac{111}{2221} = \textbf{0.049}$$

$$\textbf{Risk} \text{ of CVD death in the } \textbf{placebo} \text{ group} = \frac{189}{2223} = \textbf{0.085}$$

These numbers estimate the probability of the event (CVD death) taking place in the statin versus the placebo group. This is a population-level estimate.

Bullet Points

Relative risk (RR): the ratio of the probability of an event in one group compared to the other.

Relative Risk :

$$\frac{\text{Risk in group a}}{\text{Risk in group b}}$$

What Is the Relative Risk?

Relative risk (RR) is a ratio of the risk of an event in one group compared to the other. The **RR** of **Coronary death** in the **statin group** *compared* to the placebo group was:

$$\frac{\text{Risk of CVD death in statin}}{\text{Risk of CVD death in placebo}} = \frac{0.049}{0.085} = \textbf{0.576}$$

The result means that compared to placebo, patients with pre-existing CHD who took statin were nearly half as likely (**42%**) to die from CVD. The RR in statin was 0.576 = 57.6%, the risk reduction was 1-0.576 = .424 = 42.4%. This is the **relative risk reduction (RRR)**. Let us see a graphical example (Figure 15.3).

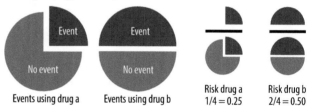

Events using drug a   Events using drug b   Risk drug a $1/4 = 0.25$ Risk drug b $2/4 = 0.50$

Figure 15.3 Comparing risk between drug a and drug b.

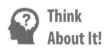

Think About It!

How would you present data of relative risk in a trial?

Four participants were treated with drug a, and a single event took place. The **risk** of an event in **drug a** was **0.25**. Another group of four were treated with **drug b**, two events took place (risk **0.50**). The **RR** of the event in the **drug a** group was *half* that of drug b and in the **drug b** group was *twice* that of group a. Participants taking **drug a** were **half** as likely to experience the event compared to participants taking drug b and participants using **drug b twice** as likely to experience the event compared to those taking drug a (Figure 15.4).

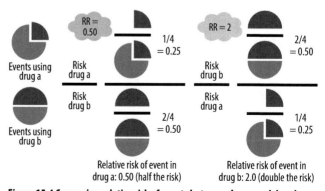

Events using drug a $RR = 0.50$ $\frac{\text{Risk drug a}}{\text{Risk drug b}}$ $\frac{1/4}{2/4} = \frac{0.25}{0.50}$

Events using drug b

Relative risk of event in drug a: 0.50 (half the risk)

$RR = 2$ $\frac{\text{Risk drug b}}{\text{Risk drug a}}$ $\frac{2/4}{1/4} = \frac{0.50}{0.25}$

Relative risk of event in drug b: 2.0 (double the risk)

Figure 15.4 Comparing relative risk of events between drug a and drug b.

Relative Risk Reduction versus Absolute Risk Reduction

It is impossible to put into context the implication of relative risk when the **underlying absolute risk** is not known. Let us examine this. Risk of coronary death was 0.049 in the statin group and 0.085 in the placebo group. We saw previously that the **relative risk reduction (RRR)** was an impressive 42%.

Bullet Points

RRR = (1-RR): relative reduction in the risk in the exposed compared to the unexposed group.

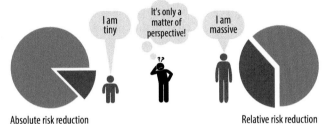

Absolute risk reduction   Relative risk reduction

Figure 15.5 Comparing relative versus absolute risk reduction using statin. RRR appears much larger but is not informative without baseline risks.

ARR = the difference in absolute risk between the two groups.

The **absolute risk reduction (ARR)** is the difference between the two risks = 0.085 − 0.049 = 0.036, **3.6% ARR**. The ARR suggests that compared to the placebo group patients who took statin had 3.6% less risk of coronary death (Figure 15.5), i.e. for every 1000 patients treated with statin compared to placebo, 36 deaths would be prevented.

Another way to describe this is the **Number needed to treat (NNT)**. NNT is the inverse of ARR. The **NNT is 1 ÷ ARR** = 1 ÷ 0.036 = 27.77. Therefore at least **28** patients would need to be treated with statins to prevent a single coronary death. Let us see another graphical example of NNT (Figure 15.6).

Absolute versus relative risk:

Up to 50% price-cut sounds attractive but is useless on its own if we do not know which items are for sale (might only be limited to £1 items!).

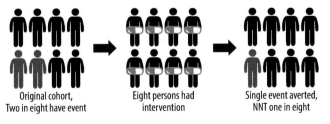

Original cohort, Two in eight have event

Eight persons had intervention

Single event averted, NNT one in eight

Figure 15.6 Number needed to treat explained.

NNT = number of patients that need to be treated to prevent a single adverse event in the treated group = **1 ÷ ARR**

Relative risk reduction appears more impressive compared to ARR. RRR is likely to give a false sense of over-estimation of the treatment effect. We can have a better idea of the size of the treatment effect by looking at the ARR or NNT [8].

NNH = number needed to harm: when the intervention is harmful it is termed NNH.

Bullet Points

OR and RR:
they are virtually similar when the outcome is rare.

OR: from zero to infinity

OR> 1 event more likely
OR<1 event less likely

Risk versus Odds in roll of a dice:

Risk of rolling a six: one in six

Odds of rolling a six: one in five

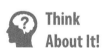

Think About It!

Is NNT absolute for different populations at risk?

Are there any other caveats when considering NNT?

Caveats in Estimating Absolute Compared to Relative Risk Reduction

Relative risk reduction is a comparison of efficacy and **remains constant** *irrespective* of event rates in the population. **ARR varies** according to the **event rate**. If we consider different studies with differing severity of disease we would get different degrees of absolute risk and ARR. ARR gets smaller as event rates get rarer in the control group.

Odds, Not Risks

Risks are not always quoted in the medical literature. Here is an example; researchers wished to investigate the cardiovascular safety of non-steroidal anti-inflammatory drugs (NSAIDs) and estimated the risk of hospital admission for heart failure. They concluded [9]:

> Current use of any NSAID [...] was found to be associated with a 19% increase of risk of hospital admission for heart failure (adjusted odds ratio 1.19; 95% confidence interval 1.17 to 1.22), compared with past use of any NSAIDs (use >183 days in the past).

Odds and risks *both* calculate the probability of an event. However, there are some important differences. In the previous example, the OR was an indication of the relative probability of heart failure-related hospital admission. The adjusted Odds ratios of 1.19 suggest that compared to a patient with a previous history of NSAID use, the probability of hospital admission for heart failure was 19% increased if the patient was a current NSAID user (OR>1, more likely).

Why Do We Have Odds in Some Studies?

There are several reasons; let us have a look. The first study was a prospective Randomised controlled study (RCT) [7]. In a prospective study, we start with a group of participants exposed to the risk factor and another group that is not exposed. We can calculate the probability of events taking place in the exposed group versus the non-exposed group

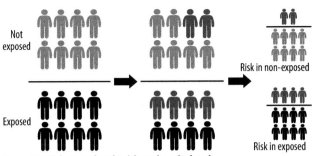

Figure 15.7 Cohort study, why risk can be calculated.

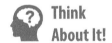

Bullet Points

Odds ratios:

Odds in group a
Odds in group b

Odds ratios can be **adjusted** for potential confounders.

Relative risk is **not** adjusted for confounders.

by observing the events (Figure 15.7). The second study was of a case-control design; cases were matched to controls [9]. Data were retrieved from a database. They identified a cohort of new NSAID users and calculated the number of cases admitted for heart failure. Each case was matched to 100 controls. We do not know the actual prevalence or exposure history. Risk estimation would have been inappropriate as discussed in the previous chapter (Figure 15.8).

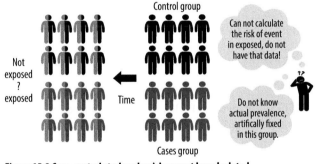

Figure 15.8 Case-control study, why risk cannot be calculated.

Think About It!

What is the advantage of undertaking a case-control study?

What would be the purpose of matching in a case-control study?

Odds Ratios: Accounting for Life's Complexities

In life, there is rarely a simple relationship between a variable and an outcome. Often there are many concurrent factors at play. Relative risk calculation can not account for confounders. With the adjusted odds ratios calculation, it is possible to adjust for the effect of confounders. Unadjusted OR is reported as crude OR in the literature. *We have previously discussed un/adjusted OR in the Bonus Stuff section of the last chapter.*

Let's turn our attention in the next chapter to a different outcome measure; time to event data analysis.

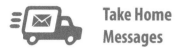 **Take Home Messages**

- Odds and risks both calculate the probability of an event.

- Risk is a measure of an outcome taking place among the whole at-risk group: number of events divided by the whole population at risk.

- Odds is a measure of an outcome taking place versus it not taking place: number of events divided by number of non-events.

- Odds ratios is the ratio of the odds in the exposed group compared to the other. OR>1 means the event is more likely. OR <1 means the event is less likely.

- Relative risk (RR) is a measure of how exposure modifies the risk of an outcome. RR is calculated by: risk in the exposed group divided by risk in the control group.

- Relative risk, if presented in isolation, is likely to over-inflate the benefits of treatment, and the underlying absolute risks should always be mentioned.

- Relative risk reduction (RRR) is the relative reduction in risk between the two groups.

- Absolute risk reduction (ARR) is the difference in absolute risk between the two groups.

- Number needed to treat (NNT) is the inverse of ARR and is the number of patients that need to be treated to prevent a single adverse event in the treatment group.

- Relative risk reduction remains constant but ARR varies according to the event rate.

- Odds and risks are nearly identical when event rates are low.

- In case-control studies, only odds can be calculated.

- Adjusted Odds ratios can control for the effect of confounders.

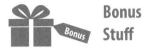

Bonus Stuff

How Absolute Risk Reduction Becomes Smaller as Event Rates Get Rarer

Let's compare the effectiveness of a magic drug M in treating migraine in a worked-out example with varying degrees of event rate (Tables 15.2 and 15.3):

	Migraine	No Migraine
Magic drug (M)	10	90
Control (C)	20	80

Table 15.2 Absolute versus relative risk reduction with a high event rate.

Risk (M): $10 \div 100 = 0.1$; Risk (C): $20 \div 100 = 0.2$;
RR in (M) = $0.1 \div 0.2 = 0.5$; RRR = 50%; **ARR = 0.2-0.1 = 0.1 = 10%**

50% RRR suggests the M group is half as likely to develop migraine compared to the C group; ARR is much less impressive at 10%.

	Migraine	No Migraine
Magic drug (M)	3	97
Control (C)	6	94

Table 15.3 Absolute versus relative risk reduction with a low event rate.

Risk (M): 0.03; Risk (C): 0.06;
RR in (M) = 0.5; RRR = 50%; **ARR = 3%**

The event rate is low; the **RRR** remains **constant at 50%** in the M group. However, the **ARR is only** 3% and less than the previous scenario due to comparatively lower event rate.

When Odds Ratios and Relative Risk Approximate Each Other

High event rate: The Odds of migraine (M) = $10 \div 90 = 0.11$; Odds (C) = $20 \div 80 = 0.25$

OR of Migraine (M) = $0.11 \div 0.25 = 0.44$; RR of Migraine (M) was 0.5

Low event rate:

The Odds of Migraine (M) = $3 \div 97 = 0.03$; Odds (C) = $6 \div 94 = 0.06$;

OR of Migraine (M) = $0.03 \div 0.06 = 0.5$

RR of Migraine (M) was also 0.5

Questions & Answers

Q: How would you present data of relative risk in a trial?

A: We have learnt that relative risk has some advantages over absolute risk because relative risk remains constant over populations, whereas absolute risk changes according to event rate. However, if we just present RR without mentioning the absolute risk this can be misleading. The best practice is to *mention both* relative risk and the baseline risk.

Q: Is NNT absolute for different populations at risk?

A: No, NNT will *vary* according to the baseline risk of the population. This is obvious when we realise that ARR varies according to the baseline risk.

Q: Are there any other caveats when considering NNT?

A: Yes, it ought to be remembered that NNT is *not an absolute* measure of the effectiveness of an intervention but an estimate of efficacy when compared to a comparator. Therefore, the comparator must always be considered. For example, when the NNT of statin is quoted, it must be stated that the NNT was assessed against a placebo treatment (at least 28 patients would need to be treated with statin to prevent a single CVD death when *compared* to placebo).

Q: What is the advantage of undertaking a case-control study?

A: When outcomes are rare and take a long time to manifest, it may be more efficient to conduct a case-control study rather than undertake a long-term prospective study.

Q: What would be the purpose of matching in a case-control study?

A: A case-control study aims to identify a potential risk factor for an outcome. However, many other variables may confound the results. The purpose of matching is to identify these variables and to select a sample where the control group and the intervention group are reasonably similar in these characteristics. Matching ensures that any difference in observed outcome between the two groups would not be due to differences in those confounding variables. It is essential to understand that matching does not control for allocation bias as the cases and controls are allocated according to the outcome status. *We have already learnt about allocation bias in Chapter 9.*

CHAPTER 16

I Will Survive!
Time to Event Data Analysis

From these considerations I have formed the adjoyned table, whose uses are manifold, and give a more just idea of the state and condition of mankind, than any thing yet extant that I know of.

Edmund Halley

Learning Outcomes

We shall discuss the following material in this chapter:
- Approach to the analysis of time to event data
- What is a hazard
- Censored data and its role in survival analysis
- Types of censoring
- How do we interpret the survival curve
- The cumulative probability of survival
- Where is the median survival time
- Why the population at risk is useful to know
- The Log-rank test: comparing survival between two different groups
- The hazard ratio and its interpretation
- The Cox regression model

Did You Know?

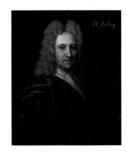

© Public domain [1].

Figure 16.1 The British astronomer **Edmund Halley FRS** (1656–1742), was one of the first to create a life table from the records of births and deaths of the population of the then German city of Breslau in 1693. The purpose of the work was to enable correct calculation of life annuities [2].

Time to Event Data Analysis: Unique Challenges

Up to now, we have discussed the estimation of continuous or categorical variables. Increasingly, analysis of a different kind of variable is of interest in the medical literature where the researchers are interested in investigating the expected duration until an event takes place. This is known as **survival analysis**; survival is the time *until* the event takes place. *Time to event data* analysis presents some unique problems. Let us see an example. Total hip arthroplasty (THA) is a widely performed and highly successful surgical procedure.

Bullet Points

Observations in time to event data analysis:

Exact: those who experience the event.

Censored: those who do not experience the event (true survival time is unknown).

Censored data is incomplete outcome data.

Example of censoring:

Not experiencing the event;

Loss to follow-up;

Withdrawal from study;

Death (when not the event of interest).

However, long-term survival for young patients varies. The researchers wished to investigate the survival of THA when implanted in patients younger than 30 years [3]. The endpoint was revision for aseptic loosening. The difficulties in data collection are immediately apparent here. Patient data were collected between 1988–2004. Participants were recruited at the time of THA and observed until revision. The risk of the event will not be the same for everyone. Patients recruited early would have had longer follow-up than those recruited late, whose ultimate implant survival may be unknown. Some patients may have died, quite a few would have moved away and may not be traceable. How do we make a valid survival analysis?

How Do We Take Account of Such Disparate Data?

To **accurately calculate** the **risk** of the *event* of interest, we need to know *when* it takes place. If we know this, our data are **exact**. If we do not know this, our data are **incomplete** or **censored**. We could opt to go for an uncomplicated analysis by only including exact data. That would mean getting rid of all patients with an unknown outcome. Although it appears to be a sound approach, we would have to reject crucial information about participants who were observed but did not experience the event, and our estimate of the population parameter would be imprecise and unreliable. It would be helpful to have a system that takes account of incomplete data.

Survival analysis allows for **censored data** to be included without affecting the integrity of data analysis. How? Let's first learn a bit more about censoring from Figure 16.2. The graph illustrates the different types.

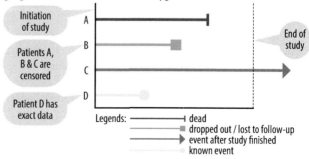

Figure 16.2 Graphical illustration of censoring in survival analysis.

Censored Data: Credit Where Credit Is Due

How do incomplete (**censored**) data contribute to data analysis? Data get credit for whatever period they provided us with information. Therefore, **patients** who are lost to follow-up, drop-off or die when death is not the event of interest, **contribute data until the point of censoring**. Similarly, patients who remain in the study but do not experience the event also contribute data. The advantage of survival analysis is that every participant contributes data; however little that might be. Censored observations are indicated in the graph by short *vertical lines* (Figure 16.3).

Kaplan-Meier Analysis: 'Survival' Until the Event

We frequently come across **Kaplan-Meier** (KM) analysis in the medical literature. It is a type of survival analysis. KM analysis aims to estimate the number of people likely to **survive** or remain free of the event of interest a given length of time in the *same* circumstances. It is displayed in a survival curve.

The event of interest may be revision surgery, cancer recurrence and is not always death. Therefore, participants 'survive' *until* they **experience** the **event**. The probability of experiencing the outcome is the 'hazard'. The instantaneous event rate in those at risk is known as the **Hazard rate**. The United Kingdom National Joint Registry database maintains up-to-date data of joint replacement implants and presents yearly analysis where the event of interest is revision surgery. The hazard is the risk of revision.

The Cumulative Probability of Survival

Here is a graphical introduction to KM survival curve (Figure 16.3). The *x*-axis is the survival time, the *y*-axis the survival probability. The horizontal line on the *x*-axis represents the survival duration in years. As soon as the event takes place, the interval is terminated, and the survival drops. The sudden downward step corresponds to the time when an event is observed. The vertical distances between the horizontal lines indicate the changes in cumulative

Bullet Points

'Survival' in KM analysis: the probability of not experiencing the event.

Survival: $S(t)$, the probability of survival up to and including time t.

Hazard: the probability of *experiencing* the event.

Hazard rate: $h(t)$, the instantaneous event rate at time t in the at-risk population.

Life table analysis: it is another type of survival analysis. The probability of the event is calculated at fixed-time points. Exact time of the event may be unknown, contrast with KM analysis where the exact time to the event is known.

Bullet Points

Survival time at the minimum follow-up time is the most accurate reflection of survival rate, as the outcome of all participants are known.

As soon as a participant is **censored** the curve becomes an **estimate**.

Numbers at risk should always be mentioned in the KM plot.

probability as time progresses. Censoring is marked on the horizontal lines with upward ticks (this function may not be available in all software). The **cumulative risk** or **cumulative probability** is the probability of an event taking place within a period. It is a *conditional* probability since the likelihood of survival up to a point is dependent on surviving up to that time-point.

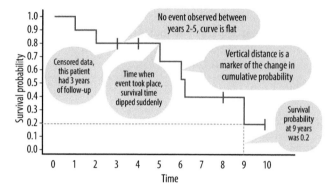

Figure 16.3 The Kaplan- Meier analysis, stair and step function.

For example, the probability of survival to year three is the probability of survival to year one times the probability of survival to year two times the probability to year three and so on. The probability of survival starts at 1.0 (100%) and falls in steps when the event happens. The dashed lines on either side of the survival plot represent the width of the CI. Median survival is the probability of survival to 0.5 (50%), which was just over six years in this plot (Figure 16.4).

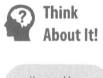

Think About It!

How would you compare survival time if there were no censored data?

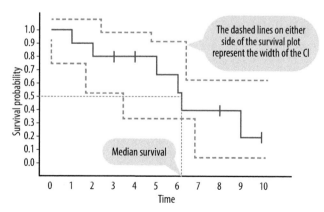

Figure 16.4 The Kaplan-Meier analysis, survival plot with 95% confidence interval.

Let's see an actual plot: below is a graph from the THA survival study and demonstrates the cumulative probability of survival of the implant (Figure 16.5) [3]. The maximum follow-up was 23 years. At year 0, the survival probability was 1.0, and at year 15 it was 0.82, so the probability of survival of THA at 15 years was 82%. Median survival is the best point-estimate for average since survival data is skewed. Median survival can *not* be calculated from this plot as implant survival did *not* reach 50% at the end of the study.

Bullet Points

Stair and step function in KM analysis:

Stair: is flat, survival estimate remains **flat** *between* events.

Step: is **steep**, survival estimate *drops* when an event takes place.

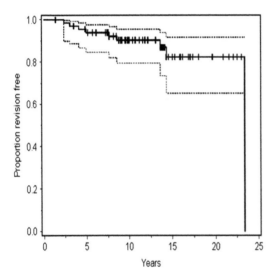

Figure 16.5 Kaplan-Meier analysis of THA survival in young patients.
© BMC Musculoskeletal Disorders, reproduced under CC BY 2.0 [3].

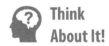

Think About It!

If survival data are asymmetric, in what direction is the skew likely in KM analysis?

Confidence Interval: Wider and Less Precise Over Time

We learnt that the dashed lines on either side of the survival plot represent the estimated 95% CI of the survival probability (Figure 16.4). The 95% CI widens as we travel in time towards the right of the plot. The widening is due to the loss of patients from the cohort. As the estimate becomes less precise, the width of the CI widens. Hence, it is best practice in KM analysis to report the population at risk (remaining cohort) along with the KM plot to enable us to assess the robustness of the survival estimate. One should also be cautious about the interpretation of the far right area of the curve where the numbers-at-risk may be low and the estimate unreliable.

When would the survival probability be zero in a KM plot?

Bullet Points

Can We Extrapolate Results Beyond Available Data?

In the study above, the maximum follow-up time was at 23 years. What if we wished to estimate the likely survival at 25 years? Is it possible? It is not possible to extrapolate data beyond the available time. There is no way of knowing the likely survival of the implant at 25 or 30 years.

Log-rank test:

it is a **significance test**. The test gives no indication of the magnitude of difference.

We need the **Hazard ratio** to calculate the difference. *We shall learn later about the Hazard ratio and how to detect the magnitude of difference.*

Survival of Multiple Groups: The Log-Rank Test

Sometimes a study involves the analysis of more than one group. If their survival plots appear different, we would be interested to know if the observed difference was significant or just by chance alone. If we did not have any censored patients and the groups were comparable, we could compare the differences with a non-parametric test (the Mann–Whitney U test). Presence of censored subjects makes the calculation complex as the groups are not comparable. In this situation, we perform the **Log-rank test**. It is a variant of the χ^2 test and compares the observed frequency of individuals who experienced the event against the expected frequency.

Here is an example; authors compared the survival of THA between patients aged <60 years or more and reported (Figure 16.6) [4]:

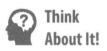

Think About It!

What is the null hypothesis of the Log-rank test in the THA survival plot?

Survival was higher in those arthroplasties implanted in patients older than 60 years, with statistical significance

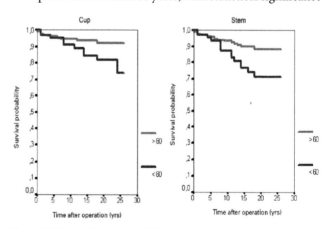

Figure 16.6 Comparison of survival plot.
© BMC Musculoskeletal Disorders, reproduced under CC BY 2.0 [4].

in the Log Rank test, both for the acetabular component (p = 0.008) and the femoral stem component (p = 0.043).

The results suggest that both stem and cup survival were more likely when implanted in patients older than 60 years compared to patients of a younger age. How can we predict what variables might be associated with implant failure? Let's consider this next.

Multivariable Cox Regression: Predicting Survival

We are interested in investigating the influence of one or more risk factors on the probability of survival. Cox regression model allows us to assess the effect of several variables on survival. High tibial osteotomy (HTO) surgery is often performed in young patients for medial compartment knee arthritis and varus malalignment. Researchers monitored patients who had HTO, the outcome of interest was revision to a total knee replacement [5]. The authors investigated the role of several risk factors including age, gender, body mass index (BMI), Kellgren-Lawrence grade of osteoarthritis, and varus angle with the Cox regression and commented:

> age had no influence on HTO survival (p = 0.32). There was no significant difference between the survival rate of men and women […] Statistical significant correlation between the preoperative Kellgren-Lawrence osteoarthritis grade >2 and HTO failure could be detected with the use of both univariate (p = 0.003) and multivariate [sic] (p = 0.01) Cox regression models.

The authors used both univariable and multivariable models to investigate the risk factors. We have learnt previously that univariable modelling is useful to investigate individual risk factors. However, the more likely scenario is that several inter-related predictors are responsible. Multivariable modelling allows for simultaneous assessment of many risk factors. Note that both categorical (gender) and numerical variables were investigated. From the analysis, we can conclude that pre-operative osteoarthritis proved to be the only significant risk factor predicting failure of HTO after adjusting for the effects of other confounding factors.

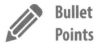

Bullet Points

Cox regression:

to investigate the effect of several risk factors on survival.

Cox regression is *multi*variable, compare with Kaplan-Meier analysis which is *uni*variable.

Both Log-rank test and Cox regression require proportional hazards assumption to be met. *This is explained in detail in the Bonus stuff section.*

Kaplan-Meier analysis in UK National Joint registry data:

National Joint Registry survival graph highlights survival estimates in *blue italics* when there are <250 implants at risk to alert the reader to the likelihood of an unreliable survival estimate.

National Joint Registry also calculates **Prosthesis Time Incidence Rate (PTIR):** this is the number of revisions per total individual prosthesis year at risk, described as number of revisions per thousand years at risk. **PTIR** helps to identify **best** and **worst** performing implants.

Bullet Points

Hazard ratio:
relative risk over time.

HR>1: risk of event increases.

HR<1: risk of event decreases.

Unadjusted Hazard ratio:
influence of a single predictor.

Adjusted Hazard ratio:
same as adjusted odds ratios, influence of a predictor controlling for other predictors.

Incidence rate (IR):
it is the number of events per unit time.

IR is described in unit of time and is the number of events ÷ sum of all follow-up time (in months/years).

Comparing Time to Event: The Hazard Ratio

The Log-rank test allowed us to investigate whether the difference in survival pattern between the two groups was statistically significant but gave no indication of the margin of the difference. We need to calculate the **Hazard ratio** if we want to appreciate the margin of difference. The hazard ratio is a ratio of the hazard rate between the two groups. Let's recall that the hazard rate is the probability of an event taking place. It is calculated by dividing the event rate at any time interval by the length of that time interval. The time interval is typically kept relatively small and thus **hazard rate**, in essence, becomes an **instantaneous event rate**. Let us see an example. Researchers investigated the predictive factors and rate of revision after Total shoulder arthroplasty (TSA) [6]. They concluded:

> Univariate and multivariable adjusted hazard rates were calculated using Cox regression analysis [...]. In multivariable analyses men had a higher hazard ratio of revision of 1.72 (95% CI 1.28 to 2.31) (p < 0.01) compared with women, and those with rotator cuff disease had a hazard ratio of 4.71 (95% CI 2.09 to 10.59) (p < 0.001) compared with patients with rheumatoid arthritis. We concluded that male gender and rotator cuff disease are independent risk factors for revision after TSA.

The authors compared the rate of revision after TSA between male and female patients and between patients with rotator cuff disease and those with rheumatoid arthritis. The Hazard ratio (HR) for men was 1.72. Therefore, men were nearly twice as likely (72% more likely) to require revision than females. The **survival probability** of TSA in men was **less**. Similarly, patients with rotator cuff disease had an HR of 4.71. They were nearly five times more likely to require revision surgery compared to patients with rheumatoid arthritis.

We have completed our learning about the analysis of different types of variables. In the next chapter, we shall learn how to assess the accuracy of a diagnostic test.

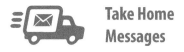

Take Home Messages

• Calculation of time to event data is complex due to differing follow-up times and variable risk of an event.

• Kaplan-Meier (KM) analysis is a type of survival analysis. 'Survival' is the length of time a participant remains free of the event of interest.

• KM analysis is an estimate of the length of time a participant is likely to survive under similar conditions. The survival function is displayed by the survival curve.

• KM analysis takes into account different follow-up times in the analysis of time to an event.

• The probability of experiencing the outcome of interest in survival analysis is the 'Hazard'.

• Participants who do not experience the event are censored. Their true survival is unknown but censored patients contribute data until the point of censoring.

• As soon as a participant is censored, the survival curve becomes an estimate.

• The survival curve has a stair and step appearance.

• The stair is the survival estimate in between events.

• The step is the drop in survival when an event takes place.

• The calculated risk of an event is the cumulative risk. It is the probability of an event happening within a period and is conditional on surviving the previous periods.

• Median survival is the probability of survival of 50% of the participants.

• Survival estimate gets less precise as patients are lost from follow-up.

• Survival estimate cannot be extrapolated beyond the end of the study.

• The Log-rank test is a hypothesis test. It compares if there is a significant difference in survival between multiple survival curves.

• The Hazard ratio is the relative risk of survival.

• The effect of confounders can be controlled by calculating the adjusted hazard ratio.

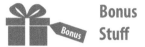

Bonus Stuff

A Worked-Out Example of Cumulative Survival

Cumulative probability of survival (to a point) is found by multiplying survival rates up to that point. We begin a trial of a new hip replacement implant with 1000 participants. At the end of year one there are 10 revisions, at the end of year two there are 20 more revisions. What is the probability of survival beyond year two?

Survival year 0 = 1000; year 1 = 990 ÷ 1000 (0.99); year 2 = 970 ÷ 990 (0.979).

Cumulative survival at year 0 is 1000 ÷ 1000 = 1. The probability of survival up to year 1 is 1.

The probability of survival past year 1 is: $1 \times 0.99 = 0.99$.

The probability of survival beyond year 2 is: $1 \times 0.99 \times 0.979 = 0.969$.

A Worked-Out Example of Incident Rate

Total number of events = 10.

Total follow-up time = 100 months.

Incidence rate = 10 ÷ 100 = 0.1 events/person month.

Assumptions that Require to be Met for a Valid Survival Analysis

Many underlying assumptions require to be satisfied for the KM analysis to be valid. These are as follows:

1. **Censoring is non-informative** and has no relation to the event of interest. The participants who were censored had the same survival probability as those who were not censored, i.e. when assessing the survival of patients after THA, an assumption has to be satisfied that those who died, dropped off the study or got lost to follow-up did not do so because they had an impending implant failure and were more likely to experience/need revision surgery (event of interest). If this was the case, then the censored population would no longer represent the population we are interested in (non-censored) and the estimation of survival probability would be biased. The UK NJR consider censoring due to death to be non-informative.

2. **Same survival probabilities**: survival probabilities are the same regardless of when the participants were recruited in the study.

3. **Proportional hazards model**: this is an assumption of the Cox regression model and the Log-rank test. The tests assume that the **hazard ratio between** the groups remains **constant** throughout the follow-up. It is *not* assumed that the hazards themselves are constant, this does vary, but the hazard ratio between the groups should remain constant. When comparing mortality after hemiarthroplasty to THA, this assumption may not be valid if patients who had THA were at higher risk of early death in the first year compared to those who had hemiarthroplasty but not necessarily so after a few years. This risk can be assessed by visually inspecting the survival plot, or by performing statistical tests [7].

Competing Risk in Kaplan-Meier Analysis

Competing risk is often present in survival analysis and may result in a biased estimate. Competing risk is said to be present when the study participant is at risk of events that may prevent us from observing the event of interest. A good example is a long-term follow-up of THA survival where patients may die before undergoing revision surgery.

A fundamental assumption of KM analysis is that patients who were censored (in this case died) were at similar risk of revision compared to patients who were not censored. This assumption may not always be valid. There is evidence that KM analysis overestimates the risk of revision arthroplasty when competing risks are present [8]. Statistical modelling has been suggested to account for competing risk in orthopaedic literature [9]. Here is an extract from a study [10]:

At 40 years, the cumulative incidence of acetabular and/or the femoral component revision or implant removal for any reason, with death accounted for as the competing risk, was 10% (95% CI 8 to 12) in female patients, and 17% (95% CI 14 to 19) in male patients.[...]

With the Kaplan-Meier survivorship analysis, the cumulative incidence of revision or implant removal for any reason at 40 years was 19% (95% CI 23 to 33) [sic] for female patients and 44% (95% CI 31 to 54) for male patients. As such, the Kaplan-Meier survivorship estimated the true incidence of revision or removal for any reason in women to be higher by 9% and higher in men by 27%. [...]

The greatest discrepancies between the competing risk model and the Kaplan-Meier models were seen in patients who have a higher annual mortality rate.

The UK NJR do not consider **death** to be a *competing risk* for survival analysis. The UK NJR survival estimate is the probability of revision assuming patient is still alive.

Questions & Answers

Q: How would you compare survival time if there were no censoring?

A: Since data are broadly non-parametric, if complete data were available, we could perform a non-parametric test. In this case, the appropriate test would have been the Mann-Whitney U test to compare the ranks of survival times between two independent groups or the Kruskal-Wallis test if we wished to compare multiple groups.

Q: If survival data are asymmetric, in what direction is the skew likely in KM analysis?

A: The probability of an event is >0, it can't be <0. Therefore, survival data in KM analysis can't be left-skewed. It will always be right-skewed.

Q: When would the survival probability be 0 in a KM plot?

A: The survival probability will only reach 0 if every patient experienced the event during the study period. In reality, since there will always be patients who have not experienced the event, the survival probability will not reach 0.

Q: What is the null hypothesis of the Log-rank test in the THA survival plot?

A: There is no difference in revision rate in THA cup and stem between patients aged over or under 60.

CHAPTER 17

High Ceiling or Low Threshold?
Accuracy of a Diagnostic Test

[..]to find out a method by which we might judge concerning the probability that an event has to happen, in given circumstances, upon supposition that we know nothing concerning it but that, under the same circumstances, it has happened a certain number of times, and failed a certain other.

Richard Price (commenting on Thomas Bayes).

  Did You Know?

 Learning Outcomes

We shall discuss the following material in this chapter:
- Sensitivity versus Specificity
- Positive and negative predictive values
- Positive and negative likelihood ratio
- Bayes' theorem and how to apply it in practice
- How to interpret the Receiver operating characteristic (ROC) curve

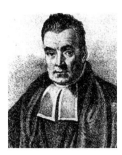

© Public domain [1].

Figure 17.1 There are no authentic surviving portraits of **Reverend Thomas Bayes FRS** (1701–1761). Figure 17.1 is widely referenced, but its provenance is unknown. He was an English Presbyterian minister who devised an algorithm for calculation of conditional probability. The work was rescued by his friend Richard Price and published posthumously by the Royal Society. His theorem teaches us how we can more precisely calculate the probability of an event when we apply our prior knowledge [2].

A Testing Time!

At the time of writing the draft for this chapter, we are deep in the midst of the Coronavirus outbreak. Everyone is understandably worried. The World Health Organisation had a simple message for fighting the pandemic: 'test, test, test'. How is testing going to help? That depends on the diagnostic accuracy of the test. When we assess the diagnostic accuracy of a test, we consider two issues:

sensitivity and specificity, what do they mean?

A real-life example may help to understand the concepts. In this security-conscious era, many of us have installed motion-activated light sensors around our property. The sensitivity of the sensor is adjustable. When the sensor is programmed to be activated at a low threshold or highly

Bullet Points

Sensitivity:
-how well the test identifies patients with the disease.

-the proportion of people with the disease who test positive (true positive rate (TPR)).

SnOUT: sensitivity to rule OUT a disease.

Specificity:
-how well the test identifies the healthy.

-the proportion of healthy people who test negative (true negative rate (TNR)).

SpIN: specificity to rule IN a disease.

sensitive mode, the detector will detect even the tiniest of movements. Small animals or even insects may trigger the sensor; it is unlikely to miss a human intruder. This is **sensitivity**, the ability to **detect** an **abnormality**.

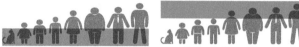

Highly sensitive motion sensor: low threshold, misses no one

Highly specific motion sensor: high ceiling, only picks adults

Figure 17.2 Sensitivity versus specificity.

If the sensor does not get activated, we can be reasonably certain (**rule out**) that there has not been a burglar intrusion. Conversely, when the sensor is activated (*test positive*), we cannot be sure that the intruder was a human (**truly positive**) and not a small animal (**falsely positive**) (Figure 17.2).

If we get fed up by a barrage of false alarms and change the setting to high, the detector will not be activated by small animals or an intrepid short-statured human intruder. This is **specificity**, the ability to be *specific* about an **abnormality**. When the sensor gets activated, we can be reasonably certain (**rule in**) that we have a human intruder. If it is *not* activated (*test negative*), the likelihood of burglary is slim (**truly negative**), but we can't be certain that a short-statured burglar has not bypassed the system (**falsely negative**).

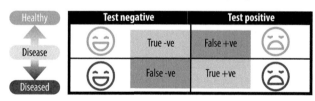

Figure 17.3 Possibilities of a diagnostic test result.

Let us now consider the example of the Coronavirus. Some individuals **harbour the disease (true positive)** and others **do not (true negative)**. The population is a mixture of these two groups of people. An ideal test would be 100% accurate and test everyone with the disease as positive (**100% true positive**) and everyone without the disease as negative (**100% true negative**). There are four possibilities when we apply a diagnostic test (Figure 17.3): (1) many patients with the disease will correctly test as positive (*true positive*); (2) some patients with the disease will incorrectly test as negative (false negative); (3) some healthy people will incorrectly test as positive (false positive); (4) many healthy people will correctly test as negative (*true negative*). What do these terms mean in context?

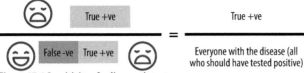

Figure 17.4 Sensitivity of a diagnostic test.

SnOUT and SpIN

When we discuss **sensitivity**, we are assessing the ability of the test to *identify the disease correctly* (Figure 17.4). We are asking how many patients with the disease are positive with the test? A *highly sensitive* test would have a low threshold and may pick up a lot of cases as positive that turn out not to be the case (**false positive**). We could not use a highly sensitive test as a discriminatory test to rule in Coronavirus since it is likely there will be *many false positive* cases. However, if one **tests negative** in a **highly sensitive** test, we could undoubtedly **rule it out** and reassure the individual.

Let's see what would happen with a highly specific test (Figure 17.5). **Specificity** is the ability of a test to be selective about the disease. We are now asking how many **healthy** individuals **test negative?** A highly specific test will have a high threshold and is likely to have cases which test negative but turn out to have the disease (**false negative**). Therefore, if the result is **positive** in a highly specific test, we can **rule in** the disease. We cannot use it to rule out the disease, as we may end up with *quite a few false negatives.*

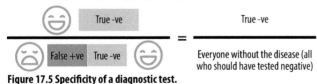

Figure 17.5 Specificity of a diagnostic test.

What is Your Preference? Depends on the Condition!

Having studied the difference between sensitivity and specificity, we now have to decide on a trade-off between a highly sensitive test (with potential for many false

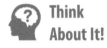

Bullet Points

Highly sensitive:

few false negatives.

Highly specific:

few false positives.

Think About It!

What is the accuracy of a test that is 100% sensitive?

How many patients would fail to test positive in a test that is 85% sensitive?

How many patients would be false positive in a 75% specific test?

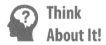

Think About It!

Which risk would you be prepared to take, more false positives or more false negatives?

positives) and a highly specific test (with potential for many false negatives) for the population with an outbreak of Coronavirus. False positive or false negative, are they equally problematic? This depends on the severity of the condition. Coronavirus can be potentially deadly, but is it better to bear the psychological trauma of a few false positives to avoid the fatal risk of a potential death (false negative)? How about the mental stress, forced isolation and financial impact of a false positive? You decide!

Do I Have the Disease if I Test Positive?

An individual will want to know, do I have the disease if I am positive? **Sensitivity** and **specificity** are **excellent** measures of the **accuracy** of the test in the **population**, but means **little** at an **individual** level. To relay this information, we need to calculate the predictive value of the test. Predictive values are indicators of the **accuracy of the positive and negative results** of the test.

A **Positive Predictive Value** (PPV) of a test is the proportion of the people with a positive test who have the disease (Figure 17.6). A **Negative Predictive Value** (NPV) of a test is the proportion of the people with a negative test who do not have the disease (Figure 17.7).

Bullet Points

The **accuracy** of a test result may **vary** depending on the Gold standard the test is compared against.

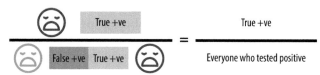

Figure 17.6 Positive predictive value.

Test **accuracy** may also **vary** depending on the **stage** of the disease. The sensitivity of serological tests for COVID-19 varies between one to three weeks of onset of symptoms [3].

Let us see an example. Researchers investigated the predictive value of rectal bleeding in screening for rectal and sigmoid polyps [4]:

Rectal bleeding had a specificity of 86%, a sensitivity of 33%, and a positive predictive value of 8% for rectal or sigmoid polyps or cancer.

Only 33% of patients with a rectal or sigmoid polyp or cancer had rectal bleeding. However, the specificity was reasonable; 86% of patients without rectal or sigmoid polyp or cancer did not have rectal bleeding. The likelihood of having rectal or sigmoid polyp or cancer provided one presented with rectal bleeding was only 8%. Although sensitivity and specificity are both inherent qualities of the test itself, the predictive values also *depend* on the *prevalence* of the disease. Therefore, PPV would be *larger* if the prevalence is *higher* and vice-versa.

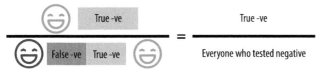

Figure 17.7 Negative predictive value.

Likelihood Ratio: another measure of test accuracy

The problem with predictive values is that they vary according to the changing prevalence of the disease. Another marker of performance of a diagnostic test is the **likelihood ratio** (LR) [5]. LR gives the same information as sensitivity and specificity but combines them into a single value. LR is the ratio of the probability of a **positive or negative test result** in a **diseased** person *compared* to a **healthy person**. LR is described in positive and negative terms. They are unitless.

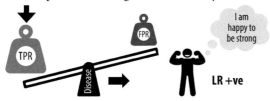

Figure 17.8 A strong positive Likelihood ratio is preferable (better detection of ilness).

$$LR + ve = \frac{\text{probability of +ve test if diseased (Sensitivity/TPR)}}{\text{probability of +ve test if healthy (1−specificity/FPR)}}$$

A **positive LR** is a likelihood of the test being *positive* in a diseased person compared to a healthy one. A higher value is, therefore, more favourable (Figure 17.8), an LR+ve of 2 suggests that for every false positive, there are two true positives. The greater the value of the LR+ve, the more likely a positive test result is a truly positive one. A **negative LR** is a likelihood of the test being *negative* in a *diseased* person compared to a healthy one (Figure 17.9). A smaller value

Bullet Points

Predictive value: what is the likelihood that the test results predict the condition, can be positive (PPV) or negative (NPV).

PPV: the likelihood of having the disease if tested positive.

NPV: the likelihood of not having the disease if tested negative.

Think About It!

Why do you think predictive values get affected by disease prevalence?

What is the screening utility of a test with an LR of 1?

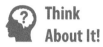

Think About It!

How would you interpret an LR+ve <1?

is therefore desirable and indicates that the test is more accurate in a healthy person than a diseased one (test is more frequently negative in the healthy). Researchers investigated the diagnostic utility of point-of-care ultrasound for pneumonia and found [6]:

> A sensitivity of 88%, specificity 86%, positive likelihood ratio 5.37, and negative likelihood ratio 0.13.

This means that a *positive* test was *more than five times likely* in someone with pneumonia than someone without. Likewise, the *negative test* was *more than seven times less likely* in someone with pneumonia.

True or made up?

'If we stop testing right now, we'd have very few cases, if any'; who said this?

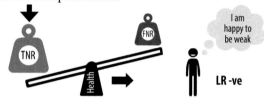

Figure 17.9 A weak negative Likelihood ratio is preferable, (better detection of health).

$$LR\text{-ve} = \frac{\text{Probability of }-\text{ve test if diseased } (1-\text{sensitivity/FNR})}{\text{Probability of }-\text{ve test if healthy (Specificity/TNR)}}$$

We can utilise LR to improve our prediction of a test result. If we know the prevalence of a disease, we can calculate its prior probability (pre-test odds), if we multiply pre-test odds with LR we get post-test odds or posterior probability. The idea of using pre-test information to reinforce or repudiate post-test probability is an important concept that stems from the work of Thomas Bayes. Let us take a look at this in more detail.

Bullet Points

Likelihood Ratio (LR): it indicates the strength of a +ve or -ve test result.

Positive LR: a *larger* value is preferable to *rule in* disease.

-it indicates better detection of disease.

Negative LR: a *smaller* value is preferable to *rule out* disease.

- it indicates better detection of health.

The Bayes' Theorem: Back to the future!

The formula for Bayes' theorem is complex, but we instinctively utilise the principle regularly in our practice. It is how we make a diagnosis from a list of differential diagnoses. Let us consider the example of two gentlemen who presented to the emergency department at the same time. They were of similar age, complained of chest pain, had abnormal ECG and raised troponin. One of them had a sedentary lifestyle with hypercholesterolaemia, the other, a fit and well marathon runner. Our interpretation of the test results would be different for these two patients. Whereas we would strongly suspect a cardiac event for the first patient, we would be less convinced for the second. In this example, we utilised the principle of the Bayes' theorem without realising it. We made a mental calculation of the **posterior** or **new** probability of a cardiac event given our **prior knowledge** of the probability of a cardiac event when one is a sedentary individual with raised cholesterol versus a fit and well person given the identical test results.

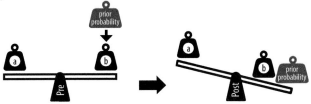

Figure 17.10 Bayes' theorem: test equally favours event a or b. Prior probability of b is higher, post-probability of b is higher than a.

Will It Rain? Bayes' Theorem to the Rescue!

We can utilise Bayes' theorem to make a more accurate calculation of the probability of an event based on previous knowledge of related events (Figure 17.10). Let us consider another example. Suppose the forecast is for a 40% probability of rain in my hometown for this weekend. Will rain spoil my weekend? Let us apply the Bayes' theorem and find out if we can calculate a more accurate probability. Given on average it rains for ten days a month and the accuracy of weather prediction is 60% when rain is forecasted, we can now calculate a more precise probability of rain for the weekend:

The probability (P) of **rain** in July (0.33)
P (rain if **predicted**) = (0.60), **predicted probability** of rain (0.40)
The calculated new **P (rain for the weekend)** = (0.33 × 0.60) ÷ 0.40 = 0.495.
There is a 50/50 chance of rain. Better have an umbrella!

Finding The Right Balance: the ROC Curve

We have learnt that there is a trade-off between sensitivity and specificity. How do we strike the right balance? When

Bullet Points

Bayes' theorem:
helps to more precisely calculate **post-test probability** of a disease.

To calculate the updated or **posterior** probability of a disease, we require the following information:

-**prior probability** of the disease (prevalence).

-**accuracy** of the test.

The ROC curve:

- plots sensitivity against false positives.

- compares different diagnostic thresholds.

Think About It!

Considering the modest accuracy of serological tests for COVID-19, what advice would you give to an anxious colleague with a negative test?

Did You Know?

The ROC curve was first developed during the Second World War to optimise radar detection and help radar operators differentiate between a bird and an incoming enemy plane. They were named 'Receiver operator characteristic'. The invention transformed aerial combat and may have helped to win the war [8]!

a test result is on a continuous scale, we can plot a graphical analysis known as the receiver operating characteristic (ROC) to compare different cut-off levels of diagnostic accuracy to choose the right balance (Figure 17.11). The ROC curve is constructed by plotting **sensitivity** against **1-specificity**. We have already learnt that **specificity** is the ability of a test to *correctly* identify a *healthy* person as *negative*. Therefore **1-specificity** is the *rest of the healthy cases who would be incorrectly* identified as *positive (false positive rate)*. It is a plot of *true positive versus false positive rate* (**TPR versus FPR**). Each point on the curve represents a specific decision threshold. Different cut-off points will affect the true and false positive rates differently, there will **always** be a **trade-off**. An optimum cut-off level is chosen depending on whether one wishes to avoid false positives or false negatives.

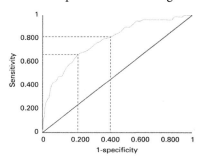

Figure 17.11 The Receiver operating characteristic (ROC) curve: optimising the test threshold.
Reproduced with permission and © of The British Editorial Society of Bone & Joint Surgery [7]. *Stippled lines are ours to indicate the different cut-off points.*

Think About It!

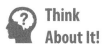

What is the predictive power of a test that lies below the diagonal line?

Can you think of a case for changing the diagnostic threshold once established?

Here is an example. The authors wished to investigate a threshold of preoperative haemoglobin that would predict the requirement for blood transfusion in patients undergoing total knee replacement surgery. Figure 17.11 shows the different choices of cut-off values, a sensitivity of 0.80 would mean specificity of 0.60, specificity would improve to 0.80 if sensitivity is curtailed to around 0.65. The authors found a threshold of 13.75 g/dl for male patients predicted a transfusion rate of 16.13% compared to 3.37% below the threshold and the area under the ROC curve for the threshold was 0.79 [8]. The area under the curve (AUC) is an overall probability of the correct prediction of the test. The range of maximum values of the AUC is between 0 to 1, 1 being a perfect test. The AUC is an index of how well the same test performs in the diseased compared to the healthy population. It is helpful to compare the diagnostic accuracy of different testing methods.

In the next chapter, we shall learn about statistical techniques to combine results from multiple studies: the 'meta-analysis'.

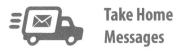

Take Home Messages

- Sensitivity is a marker of how well a test identifies patients with the disease.

- Sensitivity is the proportion of people with the disease who test positive.

- A highly sensitive test can be used to rule out a disease.

- Specificity is a marker of how well a test identifies healthy patients.

- Specificity is the proportion of healthy people who test negative.

- A highly specific test can be used to rule in disease.

- Both sensitivity and specificity are population-level parameters and not helpful for individual-level interpretation.

- Predictive value is helpful to understand the accuracy of a positive or negative test result at the individual level.

- Positive predictive value is the likelihood of having the disease if tested positive.

- Negative predictive value is the likelihood of being healthy if tested negative.

- Predictive values are affected by disease prevalence.

- Likelihood ratio (LR) is a ratio of the probability of a positive or negative test result in a diseased individual compared to a healthy person.

- A positive LR is the likelihood of testing positive if one is diseased rather than healthy.

- A larger value for positive LR indicates greater likelihood to test positive if diseased.

- A negative LR is the likelihood of testing negative if one is diseased rather than healthy.

- A smaller value for negative LR indicates greater likelihood to test negative if healthy.

- The Bayes' theorem allows a more precise calculation of the probability of disease by taking into account the pre-test probability and the accuracy of the test.

- The receiver operating characteristic (ROC) curve is constructed by plotting sensitivity against 1-specificity.

- The ROC curve is useful to compare the performance of different test thresholds.

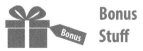

Bonus Stuff

The Formula for Diagnostic Accuracy

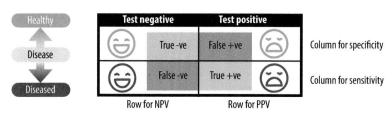

Figure 17.12 Formula for diagnostic accuracy of a test result.

$$\text{Specificity} = \frac{TN}{TN + FP \text{ (all in health)}}$$
$$\text{(negative in health)}$$

$$\text{Sensitivity} = \frac{TP}{TP + FN \text{ (all with disease)}}$$
$$\textbf{(positive in disease)}$$

$$PPV = \frac{TP}{TP + FP} \; ; NPV = \frac{TN}{TN + FN} \; ; LR + ve = \frac{\text{Sensitivity}}{1 - \text{Specificity}} \; ; LR \text{-} ve = \frac{1 - \text{Sensitivity}}{\text{Specificity}}$$

A Worked-Out Example: Diagnostic Accuracy of a Study

Let us investigate the diagnostic accuracy of a test (see Table 17.1):

		Disease positive 100	Disease negative 100	Total 200
Test positive	110	85 (TP)	25 (FP)	PPV
Test negative	90	15 (FN)	75 (TN)	NPV
Total	200	Sensitivity	Specificity	

Table 17.1 Worked-out example of the diagnostic accuracy of a test.

Sensitivity = 85/85 +15 = **85%**; **Specificity** = 75/75 + 25 = **75%**; **PPV** = 85/85 + 25 = **77%**;
NPV = 75/75 +15 = **83%**; **LR + ve** = 0.85/0.25 = **3.4**; **LR - ve** = 0.15/0.75 = **0.2**.

More about the Bayes' Theorem

The formula for the Bayes' theorem is (Figure 17.13):

$$P(A|B) = \frac{P(B|A) \times P(A)}{P(B)}$$

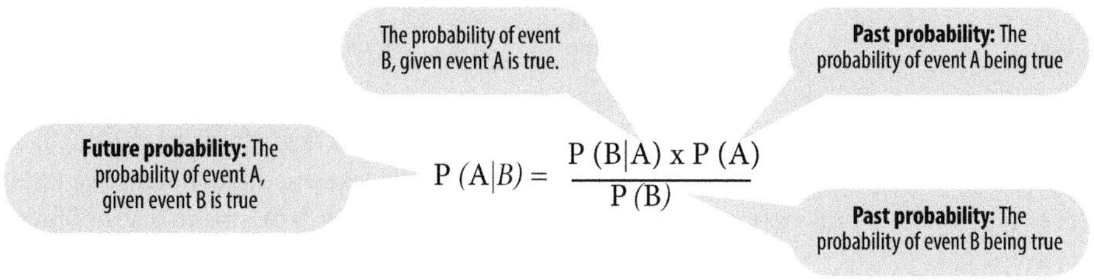

Figure 17.13 Bayes' theorem, how to better predict the future by knowing the past.

P (A|B): the probability of event A, given event B is true (has already taken place)
P (B|A): the probability of event B, when event A is true (has already taken place)
P (A): the probability of event A being true, **P (B)**: the probability of event B being true

Revisiting the example of a rainy day in my hometown,

$$P \text{ (Rain when the forecast is positive)} = \frac{P \text{ (positive forecast when it rains)} \times P \text{ (Rain)}}{P \text{ (Positive forecast)}}$$

= (0.60 x 0.33) ÷ 0.40 = 0.495 = 49.5% = a 50/50 chance of rain.

What Are the Chances I Have the Coronavirus?

Let us utilise Bayes' theorem to calculate the probability that someone with a positive test has contracted the virus. According to the current data (July 2020), around four in 1000 people may have contracted the disease in the UK. Let us assume the test has a sensitivity and specificity of 90%. We want to find out the **P (virus +ve given test +ve)**. We know that:

Prevalence = **P (virus)** = 0.004; Sensitivity = **P (test +ve given virus +ve)** = 90% = 0.90.

We need one more piece of information to complete the puzzle:

P (test +ve): what is the probability of the test being positive in the target population?

The test has a sensitivity and specificity of 90%. Therefore, the **TPR** is 0.90 and **FPR** is 0.10.

P (test +ve) = P (test +ve if disease +ve) + P (test +ve if disease -ve)

P (test +ve) = P(virus) × TPR + P (No virus) x FPR

P (test +ve) = 0.004 × 0.90 + 0.996 × 0.10 = 0.0036 + 0.0996 = 0.1032

$$P \text{ (virus +ve given test +ve)} = \frac{P \text{ (test+ve given virus+ve)} \times P(\text{virus})}{P(\text{test+ve})}$$

$$P \text{ (virus +ve given test +ve)} = \frac{0.90 \times 0.004}{0.1032} = 0.0348, \textbf{P (virus +ve given test +ve) is 0.0348}$$

If you test positive for the virus, your chance of having contracted the disease is a mere 3.48%! Why do we have such a low likelihood of disease in a highly sensitive test? Because of the low prevalence of the disease; the true positives drowned in a sea of false positives!

What if you test positive the second time? When you test positive the second time, your prior probability starts at 3.48%, so your posterior probability goes up to 0.30 or 30%. Try the calculation yourself; all the other parameters remain the same. The philosophy of Bayes' theorem is straightforward: we may not know the reality well, but we can update our knowledge as we gather more and more information. Bayes' theorem is used widely in our everyday lives. How does the search engine read your mind? It uses Bayes' theorem.

Understanding the Receiver Operating Characteristic Curve

We previously saw that 1-specificity is plotted on the *x*-axis and the sensitivity on the *y*-axis to construct the ROC curve. If we made random guesses with a coin, we would be correct in 50% of cases. The constructed curve would fall on the diagonal line (Figure 17.14).

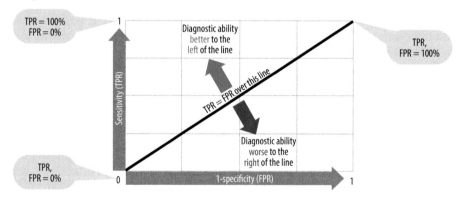

Figure 17.14 The Receiver operating characteristic (ROC) curve.

Any value on the black diagonal line cannot diagnose the diseased population correctly (TPR (0.5) = FPR (0.5)). An ideal test will have a high sensitivity and a low false positive test. A 100% accurate test will have a sensitivity of 1 and a false positive rate of 0. The upper left corner represents the best point of accuracy; both sensitivity and specificity are 100%, the closer a test to the upper left-hand corner, the better the accuracy.

Questions & Answers

Q: What is the accuracy of a test that is 100% sensitive?

A: Accuracy of a test is not the same as sensitivity. A 100% sensitive test means the test is positive in all patients with the disease, and there is no false negative case. However, this does not guarantee any false positive case will not be present. A highly sensitive test is likely to have many false positive test results.

Q: How many patients would fail to test positive in a test that is 85% sensitive?

A: A test that is 85% sensitive means out of 100 patients with the disease, 85 would test positive, and 15 would fail to test positive with the test (false negative).

Q: How many patients would be false positive in a 75% specific test?

A: A test that is 75% specific means out of 100 patients without the disease, the test would be negative in 75 of them; the false positive rate is 25.

Q: Which risk would you be prepared to take, more false positives or more false negatives?

A: The choice depends on the severity of the underlying condition. If a disease is potentially fatal, then one would be willing to risk a few false positives to avoid missing a potential death. Whereas if the disease were mild one would wish to ensure the test was very specific.

Q: Why do you think predictive values get affected by disease prevalence?

A: The predictive values are indicative of the number of positive and negative tests correctly identified as such. Even if sensitivity and specificity remain the same, changing prevalence affects the number of false positives and negatives and thus the predictive values. Here is an example (Table 17.2): disease prevalence 50% versus 5%, sensitivity 80%, specificity 75%. Population, n=100.

Prevalence 50%	Disease +ve	Disease -ve	Prevalence 5%	Disease +ve	Disease -ve
Test +ve	40	12	Test +ve	4	24
Test -ve	10	38	Test -ve	1	71
	PPV = 40 / 52	NPV = 38 / 48		PPV = 4 / 28	NPV = 71 / 72
	= 0.77	= 0.79		= 0.14	= 0.99

Table 17.2 Comparing disease prevalence and predictive values.

Q: What is the screening utility of a test with an LR of 1?

A: A test with an LR of 1 has no screening utility at all. The test result is equally likely in an individual with the disease as in the one without the disease.

Q: How would you interpret an LR+ve <1?

A: A result of LR+ve < 1 means that an individual with a positive test result is more likely to be healthy than diseased.

Q: What is the diagnostic accuracy of a test that lies on the diagonal line?

A: The diagnostic accuracy of a test that lies on the diagonal line is no better than random guesswork. The diagonal line has a value of (0.5, 0.5). The rate of TP equals FP in this test and the test is correct 50% of the time. The predictive power of a test that lies below the diagonal line is worse than that of a random guess.

Q: True or made up? *'If we stop testing right now, we'd have very few cases, if any'*; who said this?

A: True! Donald Trump, while President of the US, made this statement in a press conference while commenting on the rising Coronavirus toll in the US [9].

Q: Considering the modest accuracy of serological tests for COVID-19 what advice would you give to an anxious colleague with a negative test?

A: We know that although the pre-test probability of COVID-19 is low in the general population, it is much higher for a frontline health worker. Therefore, taking into account the pre-test probability, a negative test should be treated with caution. The correct advice would be to ask the colleague to self-isolate if he/she had strong symptoms of COVID-19. In an individual with a high pre-test probability of COVID-19, a negative test would still mean a comparatively higher risk of disease. If your colleague went back to work, there is a risk he/she could inadvertently spread the infection to vulnerable individuals.

Q: Can you think of a case for changing the diagnostic threshold once established?

A: The diagnostic threshold may vary depending on the intended use of the diagnostic test. When the test is used as a screening tool to pick up a new disease, we may wish to change the threshold and choose a cut-off value with higher sensitivity. Alternatively, when we want to use the test as confirmatory, we may want to change the cut-off value to one with higher specificity.

CHAPTER 18

Apples or Oranges?
Meta-Analysis of Selected Studies

It is surely a great criticism of our profession that we have not organised a critical summary, by speciality and subspeciality, adapted periodically, of all randomised controlled trials.

Archie Cochrane

Learning Outcomes

We shall discuss the following material in this chapter:
- What is a meta-analysis
- The purpose of conducting a meta-analysis
- Heterogeneity and the different types thereof
- How we can identify statistical heterogeneity
- Why we cannot directly add different study results together
- How studies are weighted
- How to pool binary and continuous data
- The summary statistic used in meta-analysis
- How to interpret a Forest plot
- What is a funnel plot

Did You Know?

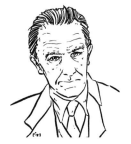

Figure 18.1 Archibald L. Cochrane **CBE** (1909–1988), was a Scottish physician but spent most of his working life in Wales. He argued for the adoption of randomised controlled trials to test treatments and to collate reliable and up-to-date evidence. His monograph *Effectiveness and Efficiency: Random Reflections on Health Services* set in motion a train of events that eventually led to the formation of the Cochrane collaboration [1].

What Is a Meta-Analysis?

Meta-analysis is a statistical technique used to **combine** the findings from **several selected studies** to provide a **single summary estimate** of the treatment effect. It is vital to appreciate the difference between a systematic review and a meta-analysis. A systematic review is a research technique used to get the answer to a specific clinical question. A **meta-analysis** is merely the **statistical section** of a systematic review. One may perform a systematic review but decide not to conduct a meta-analysis if the selected studies prove unsuitable for a summary estimate. Here is an example; the authors conducted a systematic review to assess [2]:

Bullet Points

Meta-analyis:
it is a statistical method for *combining* different studies to calculate a *single* summary estimate.

Systematic review is conducted *without* meta-analysis if studies are not suitable for providing a single summary estimate.

The **advantage of meta-analysis** is in *pooling* the results of studies to increase available sample size, reduce Standard Error, improve precision, and increase statistical power.

whether pre-operative physical factors are associated with post-operative outcomes in adult patients [≥16 years old] undergoing lumbar discectomy or microdiscectomy.

They had a specific research question and a well-defined search technique with explicit inclusion and exclusion criteria. However, in the process of critical appraisal of the retrieved studies, they concluded that available evidence was not suitable for arriving at a summary estimate. Therefore the authors continued with the systematic review but did not conduct a meta-analysis. Instead, they provided a narrative synthesis of the studies [2]:

Meta-analysis was not possible [risk of bias, clinical heterogeneity]. A narrative synthesis was performed.

Why Perform a Meta-Analysis?

Meta-analysis brings together the results of several studies to provide a summary estimate. The advantage of a meta-analysis should be clear if we recall our previous discussion about sample size and study power. **Increasing** the **sample size** helps to **reduce the Standard Error** (SE) of the estimate and increases the precision of the sample estimate. More studies usually mean more events of interest and improved statistical power of the study, reduced SE, and improved precision of the effect estimate.

Let us see an example. Authors wished to investigate if pulsed electromagnetic field therapy (PEMF) improved pain in patients suffering from osteoarthritis of the knee [3]. They were able to pool together data from five randomised controlled trials (RCTs) comparing PEMF with placebo. The combination of five trials provided 276 patients. Individually, the trials had between nine and 41 patients and were most likely underpowered to identify a clinically meaningful difference. By pooling the studies together the authors were able to more precisely estimate the treatment effect. A meta-analysis also helps us to assess and examine the consistency of effect measure across studies. If we have relevant data, we can also estimate the answer to a different clinical question than the one addressed in the primary study.

Before Pooling Studies: Assessing for Heterogeneity

Different studies inevitably come from different samples, therefore, there may be variation in the population, intervention, or results. This variation is known as **heterogeneity**.

Heterogeneity may be **clinical**, due to variation in participants, intervention, outcome etc. It may also be **methodological** due to the variation in study design. Scrutiny of the studies would allow one to judge whether clinical and methodological heterogeneity exists. Either of these may result in variation in the study results that is known as **statistical** heterogeneity. A degree of natural variation in results between trials is expected due to chance. Statistical heterogeneity is present when variation well beyond the scope of chance is present due to difference in treatment effect.

How Can We Assess Statistical Heterogeneity?

The purpose of a meta-analysis is to pool together various studies into a single summary estimate. The summation is only feasible if studies are homogeneous enough to provide a meaningful summary. If there is sufficient common ground between studies, even if individual studies are different, they would have measured the same treatment effect. In that case, we expect to observe a variation in the confidence interval of treatment effects between studies, but these should overlap. On the other hand, if there is statistical heterogeneity, there will be a poor overlap (Figure 18.2a and 18.2b).

Bullet Points

Heterogeneity:
the variation between studies.

Types of heterogeneity:

-clinical

-methodological

-statistical

Statistical heterogeneity: variation in treatment effect beyond that expected due to chance.

Chi-Squared test: to assess for statistical heterogeneity.

I^2 **statistic:** to assess the impact of heterogeneity on study results.

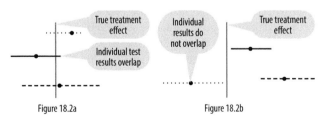

| Figure 18.2a | Figure 18.2b |

Figure 18.2a Statistical heterogeneity absent (all studies measured the same treatment effect).
Figure 18.2b Statistical heterogeneity present (studies probably measured different treatment effects).

Bullet Points

Suspect heterogeneity when I^2 statistic >50%.

Statistical heterogeneity can be explored with a **L'Abbé** plot (*explored further in the Bonus Stuff section*).

Fixed-effects meta-analysis: true intervention effect is **fixed** or the same across studies.

Random-effects meta-analysis: true treatment effect is **randomly** distributed and different across studies (but belongs to the same underlying distribution).

How Do We Calculate Heterogeneity?

We can calculate statistical heterogeneity with the **Chi-Squared test**. The test statistic is Q. Large values of Q suggest probable heterogeneity. This test is largely dependent on the number of studies. It has low power when the number of included studies is small and vice versa.

The other test is the I^2 **statistic**. It is not dependent on the number of studies. The I^2 statistic does not directly calculate heterogeneity but indicates its impact on the meta-analysis. It indicates the proportion of variability that is due to heterogeneity rather than chance. I^2 statistic value ranges from 0–100%. A value >50% indicates probable heterogeneity [4].

What Should I Do When Heterogeneity Is Present?

If heterogeneity is found to be significant authors may well choose not to continue with meta-analysis but instead provide a narrative synthesis [2]. The alternative option is to conduct a random effects meta-analysis. Here is an example; authors investigated the effect of shockwave therapy in managing rotator cuff disease with or without calcification. They selected nine studies for meta-analysis. The I^2 statistic value for reporting mean function was 79.46%. The authors proceeded with a random-effects meta-analysis [5].

Fixed- versus Random-Effects Model

Fixed-effects meta-analysis assumes that the true effect of the intervention is the same across studies. Hence if there is variability in results, this is purely due to random variation. This model does not recognise statistical heterogeneity. A random-effects model assumes that the different studies have different true treatment effects, but they all belong to a common distribution. When there is significant heterogeneity, a random-effects model may be preferable.

Can We Not Just Add Together the Trial Results?

Combining study results into a simple arithmetic average is a simple and attractive proposition, but is it feasible? Let's go back and review the previous study that assessed the role of PEMF for improving knee pain [3].

The authors finally selected five studies for meta-analysis. All the studies were RCTs and compared PEMF against placebo. So far, so good. However, on further scrutiny, we find two of the studies used low-frequency PEMF requiring long duration of treatment while three studies used high-frequency devices with shorter treatment duration. Two of the studies reported pain relief using the Visual Analogue Scale (VAS) while the other three used Western Ontario and McMaster Universities Osteoarthritis Index (WOMAC) pain scale. Three of the included studies reported functional outcome with the WOMAC physical function scale, one study used the Arthritis Impact Measurement Scale (AIMS), and the other study did not report any functional outcome. How could we possibly add together the results and make sense of it? We couldn't.

A Fair Opportunity, Not Equal Opportunity For All

There is another reason why it is not fair to add together study results. Adding together study results to calculate an arithmetic average would give equal weight to each study. This is unfair. We understand from our previous discussions that the population mean is an unknown quantity and it is estimated from the samples. We also know that SE is an estimate of how near the sample means are from the population mean. The precision of SE depends on the sample size and the sample variance. These will both vary between studies. Therefore some studies would be closer to the true population mean than others.

Giving equal weight to each study would undermine the quality of evidence generated from studies that are closer to the truth. We don't need equal opportunity; we need a system of fair opportunity. A fair system would look at the event rates as well as the variance in a sample.

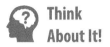

Think About It!

How would the differences between the fixed- and the random-effects model affect the calculation of the confidence interval?

Can you think of any other reason why study results should not directly be added together?

Bullet Points

A special statistical technique is used to pool together different studies. This is known as **weighting**.

Weighting takes into account sample size and variance.

Bullet Points

Inverse variance method: suitable for pooling studies with continuous outcome.

Mantel-Haenszel method: suitable for pooling studies with binary outcome.

How Do We Combine Study Results into a Single Estimate?

We achieve it by '**weighting**' studies. Weighting acknowledges the role played by studies that are likely to be closer to the truth by giving more weight to studies that have a larger sample size or more events of interest. There are several recognised techniques for pooling together of studies:

Inverse variance method: in this method, weighting is allocated in inverse proportion to the variance of the effect estimate. In other words, studies that have wider confidence interval are allocated less weight (Figure 18.3). Inverse variance method is the preferred technique for pooling together of continuous outcome variables.

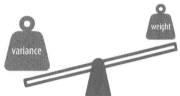

Figure 18.3 Inverse variance method: the more the variance the less the weight.

Mantel-Haenszel method (MH): this is the preferred method for pooling of a binary outcome variable. The MH method gives greater emphasis to study size but also takes into account the variance. When data or event rates are low, this method is more robust for calculation of the effect estimate.

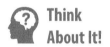

Think About It!

Can you think of a drawback of the inverse variance method?

In the spirit of fair opportunity, should a better-quality study not have more weight?

How Do We Calculate the Summary Statistic?

Continuous Outcome: Same Scale

The calculation of the summary statistic for continuous data is relatively straightforward when studies use the same scale. We can easily calculate the absolute mean difference in the same natural unit of the scale. This method is known as the **Weighted mean difference** (WMD).

Continuous Outcome: Different Scale

When studies investigate the same outcome but use

different scales, we have two options. If the conversion factor is known, we can use it to convert all to the same scale (pounds to kilograms, etc.). More often the conversion scale is unavailable. In that case, we have to calculate the **Standardised mean difference** (SMD). The SMD method uses the standard deviation to standardise the mean differences from different studies into a uniform scale. The formula is:

$$\text{SMD} = \frac{\text{Difference in mean outcome between groups}}{\text{Standard deviation of outcome among participants}}$$

The SMD method is analogous to the situation we previously came across while learning the normal distribution, where conversion of raw distribution into a Standard normal distribution allowed us to compare scores from different samples. SMD is calculated by dividing the difference in mean outcome by the Standard deviation of the outcome. Irrespective of the scales used, the SMD will be the same for studies provided the difference in the mean is of the same proportion to the standard deviation. An example is reproduced below (see Table 18.1) [5].

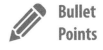

Bullet Points

Summary statistic in continuous outcome:

Weighted mean difference (WMD): when different studies use the same measurement scale.

Standardised mean difference (SMD): when different studies use different measurement scales.

Outcomes	Anticipated absolute effects* (95% CI)		Relative effect (95% CI)	№ of participants (studies)
	Risk with placebo	Risk with shock wave therapy		
Pain relief > 50%[a] Follow-up: 3 months	375 per 1000	413 per 1000 (232 to 728)	**RR 1.10** (0.62 to 1.94)	74 (1 study)
Pain Multiple scales[e] translated to VAS 0–10 (10 was severe pain)[f] Follow-up: 3 months	Mean pain in the control group was **3.02 points**[g]	Mean pain in the intervention group was **0.78 points better** (0.17 better to 1.4 better)	**SMD –0.49** (95% CI –0.88 to –0.11)	608 (9 studies)
Function Multiple scales[e] translated to Constant 0–100 scale (100 was best function)[f] Follow-up: 3 months	Mean function in the control group was **66 points**[g]	Mean function in the intervention group was **7.9 points better** (1.6 better to 14 better)	**SMD 0.62** (95% CI 0.13 to 1.11)	612 (9 studies)

Table 18.1 Summary estimate from Surace et al. [5].
© Cochrane collaboration, reproduced with permission.

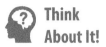

Think About It!

Authors investigated the effect of shockwave therapy in managing rotator cuff disease with or without calcification. Pain and function were reported using multiple scales. The reviewers reported the summary statistic by SMD.

How would SMD account for differences in the direction of scales, for example combining two scales where scale value increases with increased disease severity in one and reduced disease severity in the other?

Summary Statistic for Binary Outcome

When the outcome of interest is binary; risks, odds, risk difference etc. can be calculated. Both absolute difference (risk difference) and relative difference (risk or odds ratio) can be calculated. In Table 18.1 above, we observed that pain relief was dichotomised and reported as a risk ratio.

Displaying Meta-Analysis: The Forest Plot

The Forest plot is a graphical illustration method to display results of a meta-analysis. The plot contains point estimate and confidence interval for the chosen effect measure (SMD, WMD or RR, OR etc.). A horizontal line indicates the confidence interval (CI) of each trial. The square block on the horizontal line represents the weight allocated to each trial. A diamond represents the summary estimate; the ends of the diamond indicate the width of the CI. A vertical line in the middle indicates the line of no effect. If CI crosses this line, the treatment effect is not significant (Figure 18.4).

Bullet Points

Forest plot: a graphical illustration of meta-analysis.

Smaller trials have **wider CI and less weight.**

The **diamond** at the lowest row represents the **summary** estimate.

The **two ends** of the diamond represent the **confidence interval** of the **summary** estimate.

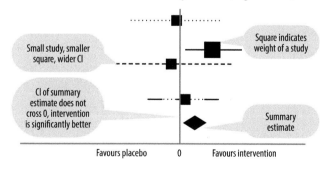

Figure 18.4 Forest plot explained.

Our journey through the maze of medical statistics is nearly over, but our discussion would be incomplete without an appreciation of how statistics are often willingly or inadvertently misrepresented in the medical literature. Let us explore this issue in the final chapter.

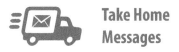

Take Home Messages

• The purpose of a meta-analysis is to pool together studies to increase sample size resulting in increased power and more confidence in the summary estimate.

• The unwarranted variation between studies gives rise to heterogeneity, which can be clinical, methodological or statistical.

• Statistical heterogeneity is present when variation in the observed treatment effect is beyond that expected due to chance alone.

• Statistical heterogeneity is calculated with the Chi-Squared statistic.

• The I^2 statistic calculates the effect of statistical heterogeneity on study results.

• The higher the I^2 value, the higher the evidence in favour of statistical heterogeneity. I^2 value of >50% is strongly suggestive of statistical heterogeneity.

• When heterogeneity is present, narrative synthesis may be performed.

• The fixed-effects method assumes that the treatment effect is fixed across studies.

• When heterogeneity is present random-effects analysis is often performed. The model assumes that the treatment effect varies across studies.

• When studies are pooled, they are weighted, taking into account the study size and variance.

• The Inverse variance method is the preferred technique for pooling of continuous outcomes.

• The Mantel-Haenszel method is the preferred technique for pooling of binary outcomes.

• The weighted mean difference is used as the summary statistic for the continuous outcome when different studies employ the same measurement scale.

• The standardised mean difference is used as the summary statistic when different scales are used.

• The summary statistic for a binary outcome is a risk or odds ratio.

• Results of the meta-analysis are presented graphically in a Forest plot.

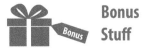

Bonus Stuff

How to Interpret the L'Abbé Plot

The L'Abbé plot is a scatterplot. It plots the outcome in the control group on the x-axis and those of the intervention group on the y-axis. The diagonal line represents the line of equality. Each circle represents a study, the size of the circle is proportionate to the precision of effect estimate of the trial. Large circles represent more precise and generally larger trials and vice versa. If intervention is better than the control, the circle will be to the left of the diagonal line and vice versa (Figure 18.5). Figure 18.6 demonstrates a real-life L'Abbé plot [6]. Authors conducted a systematic review to investigate the relationship between peri-operative adjuvant use of denosumab and tumour recurrence in the management of giant cell tumour of bone. Ten studies of varying sample sizes were included for meta-analysis. Statistical heterogeneity was explored with a L'Abbé plot. The outcome of interest was overall tumour recurrence. Risk of recurrence was higher in group 1 in seven studies, one study showed no difference and the other two showed higher risk in group 2. The outcome does not appear to be consistent. The dotted line is the line of equality and the red line represents the overall effect size which confirms a higher risk of recurrence in group 1.

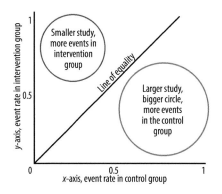

Figure 18.5 L'Abbé plot explained.

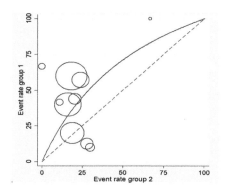

Figure 18.6 L'Abbé plot from Chen et al. [6]
© BMC Musculoskeletal Disorders, reproduced under CC BY 2.0.

A Real-Life Forest Plot

Let us refer back to the previous systematic review of the effect of shockwave (ESWT) versus placebo in rotator cuff disease. Authors assessed mean shoulder function at six weeks between the intervention and placebo and displayed the results in a Forest plot

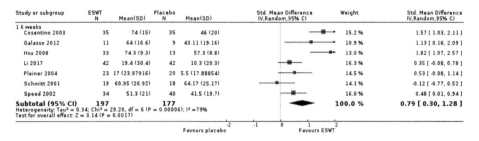

Study or subgroup	ESWT N	Mean(SD)	Placebo N	Mean(SD)	Std. Mean Difference IV,Random,95% CI	Weight	Std. Mean Difference IV,Random,95% CI
1 6 weeks							
Cosentino 2003	35	74 (15)	35	46 (20)		15.2 %	1.57 [1.03, 2.11]
Galasso 2012	11	64 (16.6)	9	43.11 (19.16)		10.9 %	1.13 [0.16, 2.09]
Hsu 2008	33	74.3 (9.3)	13	57.3 (8.8)		13.0 %	1.82 [1.07, 2.57]
Li 2017	42	19.4 (30.4)	42	10.3 (20.3)		16.3 %	0.35 [-0.08, 0.78]
Pleiner 2004	23	17 (23.97916)	20	5.5 (17.88854)		14.5 %	0.53 [-0.08, 1.14]
Schmitt 2001	19	60.95 (26.92)	18	64.17 (25.17)		14.1 %	-0.12 [-0.77, 0.52]
Speed 2002	34	51.3 (21)	40	41.5 (19.7)		16.0 %	0.48 [0.01, 0.94]
Subtotal (95% CI)	**197**		**177**			**100.0 %**	**0.79 [0.30, 1.28]**

Heterogeneity: Tau² = 0.34; Chi² = 29.20, df = 6 (P = 0.00006); I² =79%
Test for overall effect: Z = 3.14 (P = 0.0017)

-2   -1   0   1   2

Favours placebo   Favours ESWT

Figure 18.7 Forest plot from Surace et al. [5]. © Cochrane collaboration, reproduced with permission.

(Figure 18.7) [5]. The first column identifies the included studies, the second column shows the total number of participants of each trial in the ESWT arm. The third column shows the mean function (and Standard deviation) of participants in the ESWT arm at six weeks. The fourth column shows the number of participants in the placebo arm, and the next the mean function (with SD) of this group. The vertical line is the line of no effect. The results for tests of statistical heterogeneity are displayed at the lower left-hand corner of the plot (Figure 18.8). I^2 value is 79.46%, indicative of a high probability of statistical heterogeneity. The authors performed a random-effects analysis (indicated in the header of Figure 18.9). The diamond did not cross the line of no effect; the summary estimate narrowly favoured ESWT therapy.

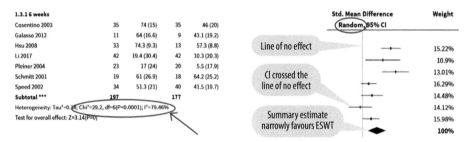

1.3.1 6 weeks					Std. Mean Difference Random, 95% CI	Weight
Cosentino 2003	35	74 (15)	35	46 (20)		
Galasso 2012	11	64 (16.6)	9	43.1 (19.2)	Line of no effect	15.22%
Hsu 2008	33	74.3 (9.3)	13	57.3 (8.8)		10.9%
Li 2017	42	19.4 (30.4)	42	10.3 (20.3)		13.01%
Pleiner 2004	23	17 (24)	20	5.5 (17.9)		16.29%
Schmitt 2001	19	61 (26.9)	18	64.2 (25.2)	CI crossed the line of no effect	14.48%
Speed 2002	34	51.3 (21)	40	41.5 (19.7)		14.12%
Subtotal ***	197		177		Summary estimate narrowly favours ESWT	15.98%

Heterogeneity: Tau²=0.24; Chi²=29.2, df=6(P<0.0001); I²=79.46%
Test for overall effect: Z=3.14(P=0)   100%

Figure 18.8 Statistics for heterogeneity.   **Figure 18.9 Results of meta-analysis.**

© Cochrane collaboration, reproduced with permission [5], (Figures 18.8 and 18.9).

The Funnel Plot and How to Read it

A funnel plot is constructed to investigate for possible **publication bias** [7]. Publication bias is present when all relevant trials are not included, as they may not have been published. The plot is useful to investigate if studies with negative effect were left out of meta-analysis. A funnel plot is a scatterplot. The *x*-axis denotes the *treatment effect.* The *y*-axis indicates the precision of *the treatment effect.* The *y*-axis is inverted, and 0 is placed on top. Included studies are plotted against **a vertical line** that represents the *pooled treatment effect,* which is the assumed true population mean.

Smaller studies are likely to be more affected by variation, have larger SE, and be less precise in the measurement of the treatment effect (further from the true population mean). These studies would be *more widely scattered* away from the vertical line of the pooled treatment effect at the bottom of the graph (where SE is larger). When *larger studies* are plotted, they will be placed *nearer the vertical line* towards the top, since these studies will be less affected by chance, are likely to be more precise in the estimation of population mean and have a smaller SE.

Since random sampling error will produce a variation in results, if our fundamental assumption that all studies come from a single underlying population is correct, and the whole spectrum of the population is sampled and results published, the plot will appear *symmetrical and triangular* due to the differences in effect estimate and SE. If there is *publication bias*, this will be evident by the presence of a *noticeable gap* in the triangle. Asymmetry in the funnel plot is not only due to publication bias, and cautious interpretation is warranted.

Here is an example [8]. Authors investigated the safety and the efficacy of open versus endoscopic carpal tunnel release via a systematic review. They constructed a funnel plot to rule out publication bias (Figure 18.10). The funnel plot below has enough data to create a pattern, is symmetrical, and there are no obvious gaps. There is no obvious publication bias.

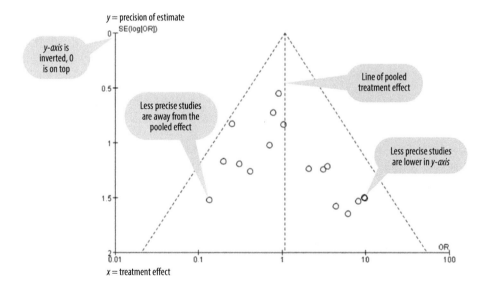

Figure 18.10 Deconstructing the funnel plot. © BMC Musculoskeletal Disorders, reproduced under the CC licence [8].

Questions & Answers

Q: How would the differences between the fixed- and the random-effects model affect the calculation of the confidence interval?

A: Since the random-effects model assumes more variation in the actual population estimate, the calculation of the confidence interval would be wider, and the summary estimate less precise.

Q: Can you think of any other reason why study results should not directly be added together?

A: When RCTs are pooled if we directly add together the study results, this will affect the benefit of randomisation and introduce confounding bias. Secondly, when included studies are of unequal size (which is often the case), simple addition is likely to give undue weight to larger studies.

Q: Can you think of a drawback of the inverse variance method?

A: In the inverse variance method, studies with small confidence intervals get allocated more substantial weight and vice versa. Such allocation is done on the presumption that the difference in variance is due to the difference in SE alone. Such is the case if all studies are part of the same population and the underlying variance is the same. If this is not correct and the difference in variance is due to a real difference in the population, then this method does unfairly undermine some studies.

Q: In the spirit of fair opportunity, should a better-quality study not have more weight?

A: Indeed, studies that are methodologically better deserve more weight. The problem is that it is difficult to find a scalar measurement technique that will justly allocate weights to studies based on their methodological quality. Therefore, in some reviews, authors decide against conducting a meta-analysis when the risk of bias is high (see the quote from reference [3], authors cited risk of bias).

Q: How does SMD account for differences in the direction of scales, e.g., combining two scales where scale value increases with increased disease severity in one and reduced disease severity in the other?

A: Standardised mean difference does not take into account differences in the direction of scales. Such a difference will have to be calculated and adjusted to ensure that the summary statistic is uni-directional.

CHAPTER 19

Lies, Damned Lies and Statistics
Untangling Facts from Fiction!

What, then, should we think about researchers who use the wrong techniques (either wilfully or in ignorance), use the right techniques wrongly, misinterpret their results, report their results selectively, cite the literature selectively, and draw unjustified conclusions?

Douglas Altman

Did You Know?

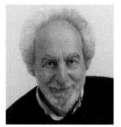

© Oxford Clinical Trials Research Unit CC SA4 [1].

Figure 19.1 'We need less research, better research, and research done for the right reasons' – this was the opening statement of the late British statistician **Douglas Altman's** (1948–2018) 1994 paper 'The scandal of poor medical research'. The paper was published in the British Medical Journal and judged in 2015 to have been the most important paper published by the journal in the previous 20 years [2].

Learning Outcomes

We shall discuss the following material in this chapter:
• How data can be manipulated to suit research evidence
• How surrogate outcomes are used to manipulate evidence
• What is p-hacking and why it is harmful to evidence-based practice
• Why one should be wary of subgroup analysis
• What do we mean by outcome reporting bias
• What the Tamiflu controversy taught us
• How industry-sponsored research can bias evidence
• How confirmation bias can affect our interpretation of results

How a Pair of Gloves Became Two

At the time of writing this book, the Coronavirus epidemic has put an enormous strain on every aspect of our life. The epidemic has tested the resolve and resource of every country in the world. The UK health authorities proved more than equal to the task, with their daily briefings and bandying about of numbers, a thousand here, a million there and a billion somewhere else. When the government was criticised for lack of provision of personal protective equipment (PPE), they came up with some numbers: they had distributed a billion pieces of PPE for frontline workers, hard to argue with that number, isn't it? Unfortunately, it later turned out that to arrive at this billion-number figure, the government machinery counted a single glove as a piece of equipment [3]. A pair of gloves became two pieces of PPE!

Such brazen display of charade with numbers perfectly illustrates the reason why the fear of 'lying with numbers' has reached such heights of infamy. As physicians with an amateur interest in medical statistics, we must appreciate that numbers have both their strengths and weaknesses. The power of a number is that it is a robust and irrefutable piece of evidence that we cannot ignore. The liability lies in how we present it. For the physician, the key utility of learning medical statistics is to be able to appreciate published evidence. Therefore, the learner should be familiar with the caveats of data manipulation. We shall not discuss gross research misconduct and straightforward mistruth. Nor shall we discuss pure methodological bias that may affect the results. We shall not discuss sample size calculation issues and errors related to the early termination of studies since they have already been discussed in the earlier chapters. Instead, we shall discuss how authors can manipulate valid data to affect research evidence. We shall explore these areas as we travel through each stage of the conduct of a trial.

The Planning of a Trial: Surrogate Outcome

When we conduct a trial, we are interested in hard clinical outcomes to assess the effect of an intervention. However, hard clinical outcomes take time to manifest and may not be observed frequently. Therefore, we may need an expensive and time-consuming trial to demonstrate a meaningful clinical benefit. In such scenarios, researchers often choose to concentrate on a physical sign or a laboratory marker as a substitute for a hard clinical end-point. Such a clinical sign or bio-marker is a surrogate marker or surrogate outcome. A **surrogate outcome** may be a causative factor or a correlated factor or a biomarker of the disease. It is expected that improvement in a surrogate marker would predict improvement in clinical outcomes (Figure 19.2). Examples of surrogate markers include tumour shrinkage as a marker of cancer survival or a reduction in serum cholesterol as a marker of prevention of cardiovascular disease. Surrogate outcomes offer useful insight into disease progression or

Bullet Points

Surrogate outcome: it is not a direct clinical outcome, a related clinical feature or biomarker expected to mirror clinical improvement.

Examples of surrogate outcome and (primary end-point):

-**CD4** count in **HIV** (AIDS-related complications).

-**Intraocular pressure** in **glaucoma** (loss of vision).

Bullet Points

Cardiac Arrhythmia Suppression Trial (CAST): the trial compared antiarrhythmic drugs to placebo in management of arrythmia after myocardial infarction. Death rate was higher in the intervention arm [7].

Anti-arrhythmic drugs had been approved on the expectation that they would improve mortality rates by preventing arrhythmia.

Data dredging: trawling through the data in order to find a suitable p-value.

drug action and are regularly investigated in research. Unfortunately, there is no guarantee that improvement in surrogate markers will translate into an improvement in clinical outcome. The clinical outcome may be affected by other biological processes, and the intervention may also affect other biological processes that, if not monitored, may result in harm. It is recommended to undertake post-marketing studies to monitor the long-term outcome of treatments borne out of surrogate outcome studies.

Unfortunately, evidence suggests that once the drugs are approved, such studies are not regularly performed [4]. Therefore, the efficacy of the drug remains unproven. There is now a large body of evidence that proves that the promise of benefit shown in surrogate outcomes often does not translate into beneficial clinical end-points [5]. Several drugs that were approved based on improvement in surrogate outcomes later turned out to be harmful [6].

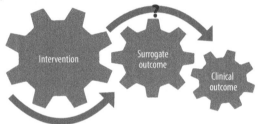

Figure 19.2 Relation between clinical and surrogate outcome.

Analysis of a Trial: P-Hacking

Correct citation of p-value:

When a significance test is performed, report the test statistic along with the actual p-value and the degrees of freedom.

Statistically significant results are attractive, for readers as well as researchers. In the hope of getting an attractive result, a researcher may continue to perform statistical tests until one comes through. This practice is known as **p-hacking**. When we reject the null hypothesis at a p-value of <0.05 there is a 1 in 20 chance that we might be mistaken. The more we repeat a significance test, the more frequent our chances of committing a type I error. Appropriate statistical corrections should be undertaken to account for this risk but may not always be done. Besides, the corrections are not fool-proof and the best option is to limit hypothesis tests only to the appropriate ones. There have also been calls to move away from the binary of statistical significance to a consideration of effect size to combat this practice of p-hacking [8].

Analysis of a Trial: Subgroup Analysis

Another technique employed by researchers to find a suitable p-value is to reanalyse primary trial data by dividing the study participants into subgroups of participants to compare treatment effect: **subgroup analysis**. There is evidence that subgroup analyses are mostly performed when primary outcome findings do not show any significant difference. The practice has been compared to a 'fishing expedition', a leap in the hope of catching something positive. There is undoubtedly a role for subgroup analysis, especially when the sample is heterogeneous, and it is plausible that treatment effect may differ in subgroups of participants. However, such analysis should be justified by clinical observation and pre-specified in the study protocol. From our previous discussion of the principles of randomisation, the *perils* of even *planned* subgroup analyses should be obvious. They are observational, and subgroups are not randomised. Therefore, the risk of confounding bias is very high [9]. They are also more likely to be affected by the play of chance. Unfortunately, a reasonably large number of subgroup analyses are performed in published papers, increasing the risk of a type I error [10]. The analyses are generally underpowered, so the risk of a type II error is also high. Available evidence suggests that subgroup analyses are mostly not pre-specified, are performed inappropriately, and analysed incorrectly, mainly to generate a suitable p-value to help publication [11]. There are plenty of examples where a headline-grabbing subgroup analysis later turned out to be incorrect [12].

Bullet Points

The deadly red dice! A planned subgroup analysis of the trial of (rolling) DICE therapy in *acute stroke* indicated that red dice increased the odds of death by 9% [13].

Born under the wrong star! The *International Study of Infarct Survival 2 (ISIS-2) trial* found that aspirin reduced overall mortality after heart attack but increased mortality in patients born under Gemini and Libra signs [10].

How to Approach and Interpret Subgroup Analyses

We should not accept the p-value as the sole evidence of treatment effect when we come across subgroup analyses. Instead, we should perform a test of interaction to confirm that the treatment effect differed across different groups. Even when the p-value is low and indicates a difference in treatment effect across different groups, the result can still be misleading. If the sizes of samples between subgroups vary considerably, this will affect the p-value [14]. Researchers have proposed several criteria when assessing the results of subgroup analyses [15]. These criteria compare the results in the context of the design, analysis, and background of

Bullet Points

Outcome reporting bias:

when a pre-specified outcome is modified or not reported or an outcome not previously specified is reported.

Outcome reporting bias in numbers [18–20]:

Statistically significant results are **twice** as likely to be reported.

A **third** of Cochrane reviews had at *least one* trial with *high suspicion* of outcome reporting bias.

Around **20%** of outcomes in primary trials may suffer from outcome reporting bias.

Treatment effect may be overestimated by **20%** due to outcome reporting bias.

the trial. The most important issue when interpreting the conclusions from a subgroup analysis is to be mindful that the results are more likely to be affected by chance.

Reporting of a Trial: Selective Reporting

On completion of a trial, after the results are correctly analysed, researchers occasionally elect to withhold specific outcomes from reporting. They may also opt to add additional outcomes that had not been originally intended to be investigated or modify an outcome from the initially intended ones [16]. Such selective reporting may be justified at times, for example, when performed before data unmasking or later, when the outcomes are judged to be redundant, or if advised by reviewers [17]. **Outcome reporting bias** occurs when authors selectively omit/modify/add an outcome based on the direction of statistical results. This practice is relatively common, and authors often resort to it without realising it [18]. Chan and Altman estimated a 20% rate of outcome reporting bias in primary trials [18]. Another review estimated that only around 13% of trials reported results correctly [19]. Lack of statistical significance is one of the most frequent reasons for not reporting outcomes, although it is not the sole reason [18]. Researchers have estimated that statistically significant outcomes are twice as likely to be reported than non-significant results [18]. Such bias matters because it results in an inflated and flawed estimate of treatment effect. Furthermore, if the authors report outcomes solely based on statistical significance, the reported outcomes may not represent the outcomes that matter from a patient and physician perspective. Reporting bias is further compounded when such evidence is collected and synthesised in systematic reviews, thus reinforcing skewed evidence [20].

Several major journals now require trials to be pre-registered, protocols published, and made publicly available to avoid or reduce the risk of reporting bias [17]. The International Committee of Medical Journal Editors has called for individual patient data to be made available for external scrutiny and validation as a requirement for publication of trials [21]. Statistical tools have also been developed for systematic reviewers to identify and adjust for missing data due to outcome reporting bias [22]. Researchers have also set up the COMET initiative to create consensus on the minimum set of outcomes to be reported in a specific clinical area [23].

Reporting a Trial: Withholding Trial Results

On other occasions, researchers may elect not to publish the results of a trial that was designed and conducted appropriately and data duly collected and analysed correctly. Such practice is especially common in industry-sponsored trials, especially if the results are deemed to conflict with commercial interests. There is no better example of this phenomenon than that of oseltamivir, popularly known under the brand name of Tamiflu [24]. Oseltamivir is an antiviral medication and is available in an oral formulation. It is a neuraminidase inhibitor that acts to competitively inhibit the virus' neuraminidase enzyme. Thus, the drug prevents new virus particles from being released. The Swiss multinational company Hoffmann La Roche developed this drug. It is indicated for treatment and prophylaxis of influenza A and B. The drug received FDA approval in 1999 but came to prominence in the wake of the Avian influenza epidemic in 2004 when governments around the world started competing against each other to stockpile this drug. Initial evidence appeared to justify this decision. A Cochrane review in 2006 had found that Tamiflu had an apparent beneficial effect in managing symptomatic seasonal flu, in the alleviation of symptoms and prevention of lower respiratory tract complications. The conclusion was based on a pooled analysis of industry data that had not been verified independently. When reviewers approached Roche for access to unpublished data, a saga ensued that is still being played out to this day.

Roche eventually relented and released data when their competitor Glaxo Smith Kline did so in 2013. An updated review based on newly available data concluded [25]:

> In treatment trials on adults, oseltamivir reduced the time to first alleviation of symptoms by 16.8 hours (95% confidence interval 8.4 to 25.1 hours, P<0.001). There was no effect in children with asthma, but there was an effect in otherwise healthy children (mean difference 29 hours, 95% confidence interval 12 to 47 hours,

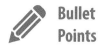

Bullet Points

The Tamiflu saga [24]:

1999: FDA approves Tamiflu.

2004: Avian flu outbreak.

2005: UK and US stockpiles Tamiflu.

2006: Cochrane review finds Tamiflu is beneficial.

2009: Swine flu pandemic.

2013: Trial data released by GSK and Roche.

2014: Updated Cochrane review finds insufficient evidence to support Tamiflu use in influenza.

2017: WHO downgrades Tamiflu from core to complementary list of essential medicines.

Global spending on Tamiflu by 2014 was **$9 billion.**

Most of the Tamiflu stockpile has **never** been used.

Bullet Points

The case of Vioxx:

Rofecoxib (Vioxx),
a COX 2 inhibitor was
marketed by Merck in
1999 as a safer alternative
to NSAID medication.

Early research raised concerns
regarding cardiovascular
safety but were ignored.

Subsequent Merck-sponsored
VIGOR study confirmed
increased risk of MI associated
with rofecoxib use but the
risk was downplayed in the
published results in 2000.

Mounting evidence forced
Merck to eventually
withdraw Vioxx in 2004.

Millions had consumed
the drug in the interim.

Estimated death toll from
Vioxx stood at 38,000
in the US alone.

In 2007 Merck agreed to a
pay **$4.85 billion** to end
all related lawsuits [28].

P=0.001). In treatment trials there was no difference in admissions to hospital in adults (risk difference 0.15%, 95% confidence interval −0.91% to 0.78%, P=0.84) and sparse data in children and for prophylaxis.

The study raised further concerns regarding complications of treatment. The World Health Organisation changed its position following the review and recommended Tamiflu only for use in severe illness in critically ill patients with confirmed virus infection. Unfortunately, public health agencies continued to stockpile Tamiflu irrespective of the updated evidence synthesis, justifying their decision to do so based on industry-funded observational studies.

The Tamiflu saga brought into the open the need for trial transparency and open data. From 2013 the British Medical Journal has espoused an **Open data** campaign under whose remit a trial will only be published if authors agree to make suitably anonymised patient data available on request [26]. The **AllTrials** campaign has called for the results of all past and present trials to be reported [27].

Conducting a Trial: Industry-Sponsored Research

The Tamiflu saga highlighted the role industry-sponsored research plays in generating biased research evidence. There is no doubt that the role of industry is welcome and is integral in the continuation of research output. However, there is evidence, as we just saw in the last section, that quite often truth becomes the casualty when there is a conflict of interest between commercial profit and research evidence. Companies have financial interests in the research they sponsor since the results will dictate whether their drug will be approved or not. We know that industry-sponsored trials are more likely to report a positive result [29]. This is true both for medicine as well as surgery and is equally applicable for observational or randomised trials [30]. The trend is also evident in company-sponsored direct comparisons of their inhouse drugs, where the drug that has the greater commercial potential is usually favoured [31].

Interpreting Results: Confirmation Bias

The twist in the tale of evidence-based medicine is that even when evidence is valid, we may have a problem accepting it due to our own inherent **cognitive bias**. Cognitive bias affects every aspect of our behaviour and interaction with society. Social science studies have shown that cognitive bias affects how voters interpret the message from prospective election candidates, how they interpret the evidence and act on it [33].

It is widely appreciated that cognitive bias can result in medical errors [34]. However, the role cognitive bias plays in the misinterpretation of scientific evidence has not received enough attention. Let us concentrate on a type of cognitive bias, confirmation bias.

Confirmation bias occurs when we seek out and favour evidence that confirms our prior belief but ignore information that is contrary to it. Such behaviour is also known as **cognitive dissonance**. Researchers have found that biased research interpretation is more common than perhaps acknowledged [35]. Recent research has also uncovered a type of biased research interpretation that has been termed 'citation distortion' [36].

Citation distortion occurs when a researcher gives undue weight and citation to evidence that favours the researcher's belief but ignores evidence to the contrary, thus creating a network of unfounded authority via biased citation. An apparent reason for citation bias is our old foe statistical significance. A meta-analysis found that statistically significant results are nearly twice as likely to be cited than non-significant results [37]. Sadly, citation bias appears to be more prevalent in the biomedical sciences compared to other disciplines of science.

This is a brief introduction to some of the caveats you should consider while assessing statistical inferences in the published literature. Our journey in the print comes to an end here but before you move on to the online section take a look at Glossary next.

Bullet Points

Researchers in the US sampled a selection of voters in 2009 who already believed in a link between Saddam Hussein and 9/11 [32].

These voters were offered evidence for and against the link and subsequently interviewed.

It turned out that the evidence had mostly made no dent in the voters' prior belief.

The respondents justified the then ongoing war against the Iraqi regime based on their belief.

Authors termed this '**inferred justification**', a post-hoc attempt to make sense of the existing reality.

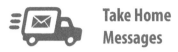

Take Home Messages

• Researchers may employ diversionary techniques to enable them to achieve desirable statistical conclusions.

• A surrogate outcome is not a direct clinical outcome but a related clinical feature or biomarker that is measured instead of the primary outcome measure.

• Improvement in surrogate outcomes does not necessarily translate into an improvement in the clinical outcomes of interest.

• P-hacking is the practice of data manipulation and continuation of statistical tests until a significant p-value is found.

• Subgroup analyses should be cautiously interpreted as they are at high risk of committing both type I and type II errors.

• Subgroup analyses should be pre-specified in the study protocol.

• Selective outcome reporting gives rise to outcome reporting bias when an outcome is selectively omitted/modified/added based on the direction of statistical significance.

• Statistically significant results are twice as likely to be reported compared to non-significant results.

• Industry-sponsored and academic research is plagued by selective reporting, manipulation and withholding of study results when the results do not favour commercial or other competing interests.

• Due to the influence of confirmation bias, we tend to favour and accept evidence that supports our preconceived beliefs.

• Confirmation bias in scientific literature has given rise to the practice of citation distortion, whereby research that favours the researcher's belief is given undue prominence and citation resulting in a network of undue authority.

GLOSSARY

Absolute risk reduction: the reduction in absolute risk between the exposed group and the unexposed group.

As-treated analysis: a type of analysis where study participants are analysed according to the treatment they received and not according to the original study allocation.

Bayes' theorem: a mathematical formula to help calculate the precise probability of an event by taking into consideration the probability of past related event/s.

Bias: a systematic tendency to deviate from the true estimate of the effect of treatment. Due to the error in the conduct or analysis of a study, the results unduly favour one arm of the study and make it look consistently better or worse than the other.

Box and Whisker plot: a graphical method of presentation of data, also known as the Box plot, commonly used to describe data that are not normally distributed.

Case-control study: a type of study where the cases are identified which have a condition of interest, a control group is selected which does not have the condition and both groups are reviewed retrospectively to compare past exposure to assess with the condition.

Censored: a participant in a time-to-event data analysis whose outcome is unknown (did not experience the event, or lost to follow-up or died).

Central limit theorem: a fundamental principle of statistics that dictates that the distribution of the means from multiple samples will follow the normal distribution even if the samples themselves do not.

Clinical significance: when the observed difference in magnitude in a study is clinically relevant.

Confidence interval (CI): reflects our uncertainty regarding the true but unknown population mean. It represents a range of probable values with an upper and a lower limit within which we expect to find the true population mean with varying degrees of certainty. 95% CI is most commonly used.

Confirmation bias: an inherent human trait whereby we tend to actively search for and give credence to evidence that appears to support our prior belief.

Confounding factor: a variable that is related to both the independent and the dependent variable in a study. A confounding factor may or may not be measured. Confounding bias may affect the results of a study if they are not equally distributed between the intervention and the control arms of the study.

Correlation: it is a statistical relationship between two random variables. Correlation indicates the extent to which the variables change in relation to each other. This does not imply causality. This relationship may or may not be linear.

Cumulative risk or cumulative probability: the probability of an event happening within a certain period of time in survival analysis. It is a conditional probability and depends on not having experienced the event up to that time.

Data dredging: to repeatedly analyse data in an attempt to find a statistically significant finding. It is unreliable as the results could be affected by both type I and II errors.

Degrees of freedom (df): the number of observations in data that are free to vary when a statistical calculation is being performed.

Descriptive statistics: the branch of statistics that helps to summarise and present collected data.

Distribution: a frequency curve showing the probability distribution of a variable.

Double-blind trial: a type of trial where the care-givers and the participants are unaware of the allocated intervention of the trial participant.

Equivalence trial: a type of trial design where an intervention is investigated to assess whether or not it is equivalent to an existing treatment within a margin of MCID.

Exposure: the independent variable that is investigated to assess its effect on the dependent variable in a study. Exposure is only observed in observational studies but not allocated. In interventional studies, the exposure is assigned by the researcher.

Forest plot: a graphical plot to illustrate summary results from pooled studies in a meta-analysis.

Hazard: the probability, in survival analysis, of experiencing the event of interest.

Heterogeneity: refers to variation between studies in a meta-analysis. It can be clinical due to differences in population, intervention or outcome; or methodological due to the variation in study design. If heterogeniety affects the results this is evident in statistical heterogeneity.

Inferential statistics: the branch of statistics that helps us to make inferences from the collected data about the population at large even though we may not have observed the whole population.

Intention to treat analysis (ITT): a type of statistical analysis of the trial results that analyses trial participants according to their original allocation and not according to the received intervention. The advantage of ITT is that it maintains the original randomisation. ITT is also a pragmatic analysis and shows the likely population-level outcome of an intervention in real life.

Interquartile range (IQR): the range between the upper quartile (Q3) and the lower quartile (Q1) of a sample and contains the middle 50% of data. IQR = Q3-Q1.

Mean: arithmetic mean is the arithmetic average of a sample; this is not the same as the geometric mean.

Median: the middle value of a sample when the values are arranged in order.

Meta-analysis: combining different studies to calculate a single summary estimate.

Minimal clinically important difference (MCID): the smallest meaningful margin of clinical benefit/harm in a study.

Mode: the most frequent value of a variable.

Negative likelihood ratio: the likelihood of a test being negative in a person with the disease compared to a healthy person.

Negative predictive value: the proportion of people tested negative that are healthy.

Negative skew: data distribution where the tail is on the left side of the curve due to the outliers being smaller than the mean. The bulk of data lie to the right of the mean.

Nocebo effect: when a placebo agent in a trial shows adverse effects. The adverse effect is known as the Nocebo effect.

Nominal: a type of categorical variable where values have no order, i.e. eye colour.

Non-inferiority trial: a type of trial design where an intervention is investigated to assess whether or not it is non-inferior to an existing treatment (could be similar or better, not worse).

Normal distribution: a type of symmetrical data distribution of a continuous random variable where mean, median and mode are identical or nearly so and placed in the centre, also known as 'Gaussian' or bell-shaped distribution.

Null hypothesis: an assumption whereby we accept that unless there is evidence to the contrary, there is no significant difference between the different treatments.

Number needed to harm (NNH): the number of patients that need to be exposed to an intervention to observe a single adverse event taking place in the exposed group. The larger the NNH, the safer the intervention.

Number needed to treat (NNT): the number of patients that need to be treated to prevent a single adverse event in the treated group. The smaller the NNT, the more effective the intervention.

Odds: the probability of an event taking place in a population. Odds are the ratio of the probability of the event taking place versus it not taking place.

Odds ratios: the ratio of the odds of an event in the exposure group compared to the control. OR>1 means the event is more likely, OR<1 means the event is less likely.

Open-label trial: a trial where the participants are not blinded.

Ordinal: a type of categorical variable where values have an order, i.e. disease severity.

Outcome: the end-result of a study, an effect measure of interest for the researchers. Depending on the variable of interest it can be an event (alive/dead), a difference (difference in a patient-reported outcome), an association etc. A study will usually have a single primary outcome that is the most important measure in the study. Sample size calculations are based on the margin of difference of the primary outcome. A study often has several secondary outcomes. Secondary outcomes are also useful measures of the impact of an intervention but they are not deemed as important as the primary one.

Outcome reporting bias: when the pre-specified outcome is not reported or modified or outcome not previously specified is reported to make the results look more attractive.

Outlier: an outlier is an extreme value in a sample in either direction, i.e. too small or too large.

Percentile: a measure of data spread, percentile divides data into 100 equal groups. Twentieth percentile means 20% of data are below and 80% above this threshold.

Per-protocol analysis: a type of analysis where only the outcome of those participants who adhered to the original intended allocated intervention is analysed (drop-outs or crossovers are ignored).

Placebo: an inert chemical substance or physical intervention without any known therapeutic benefit or harm.

Placebo effect: the beneficial effect observed in a trial in the participants who were administered the placebo agent. This is due to a combination of the natural history of the disease, regression to the mean phenomenon and patient expectation.

Poisson distribution: a type of data distribution that is observed in continuous, discrete data.

Population: everyone who has the variable of interest.

Positive likelihood ratio: the likelihood that a test is positive in a diseased person compared to a healthy one.

Positive predictive value: the proportion of people tested positive who have the disease.

Positive skew: a type of data distribution where the tail of the data is on the right side of the curve due to the outliers being larger than the mean. The bulk of the data remains on the left.

Power: the probability that an experimental study will reject the null hypothesis correctly.

P-value: the probability that a margin of difference similar to or larger than that observed in a study could be due to chance alone.

Quartile: a point that divides a sample into four equal parts with a quarter of the scores in each quartile.

Randomisation: a method of participant allocation where the probability of allocation to either the intervention or the control arm is dictated solely by chance.

Range: the range is the difference between the highest and the lowest values of a variable.

Regression: a statistical analysis method to estimate the relationship between a dependent variable and one or more independent variables. It can be linear or logistic.

Relative risk: the ratio of the probability of an event taking place in the exposed group compared to the control group.

Residual: the difference between the expected value and the observed value when conducting a statistical test. When conducting a linear regression analysis, the residual is the vertical distance from a data point to the regression line.

Risk: the probability of an event taking place in a population.

Sample: a chosen section of the population that may or may not be representative of the population of interest.

Sample size calculation: a statistical technique whereby one can determine the minimum sample size required in a study under the best-case scenario to detect a statistically significant difference if that difference does exist.

Scatterplot: a graphical method to display the value of two numerical variables using a collection of points. One variable is represented in the horizontal axis, typically noted the x-axis and the other in the vertical axis, typically noted the y-axis.

Sensitivity: the ability of a diagnostic test to correctly identify the diseased individuals.

Skewed distribution: asymmetrical data distribution with a long tail on either side due to outliers.

Specificity: the ability of a diagnostic test to correctly identify healthy individuals.

Standard deviation (SD): a measure of data spread. SD is an average measure of the extent to which individual data varies from the mean. SD is the square root of variance.

Standard error (SE): a measure of the variability of an estimate, most commonly calculated for the mean. SE is a measure of the precision of the sample mean compared to the population mean. SE is obtained by dividing SD by $\sqrt{n}$.

Statistically significant: when the results of a hypothesis test suggest there is less than 1 in 20 probability (for a threshold of $p<0.05$) that the observed differences could be due to chance alone.

Subgroup analysis: when study analysis is repeated among subgroups of participants, often in an attempt to find a statistically significant finding. Subgroup analysis is a valid tool if planned a priori.

Surrogate outcome: this is not a direct clinical outcome but a related clinical feature or biomarker that is expected to mirror clinical improvement. It is often measured instead of clinical outcome.

Test statistic: a test statistic is the numerical summary of the data from a sample that is used to test the null hypothesis. This differs according to the hypothesis test performed.

Type I error: error committed in a hypothesis test by incorrectly rejecting a null hypothesis when it is not false (false positive).

Type II error: error made by incorrectly accepting a null hypothesis when it is false (false negative).

Variable: a measurable characteristic of interest. Variable may be independent or dependent. The independent variable is the one whose effect is observed in a study. The dependent variable is observed in a study to assess if it is affected by, or has any relation to, the independent variable.

Variance: the sum of the squared differences of individual values from the mean divided by n-1. Variance is indicative of the variability of data values.

Weighting: a technique used to pool different studies together. Sample size and variance are taken into consideration when weighting pooled studies in a meta-analysis.

INDEX